HEALTH
REFORM
WITHOUT **SIDE EFFECTS**

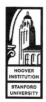 The Hoover Institution gratefully acknowledges
the following individuals and foundations
for their significant support of the
Working Group on Health Care Policy
and this publication:

LYNDE AND HARRY BRADLEY FOUNDATION

THE HEALEY FAMILY FOUNDATION

HEALTH REFORM

WITHOUT **SIDE EFFECTS**

MAKING MARKETS WORK FOR INDIVIDUAL HEALTH INSURANCE

MARK V. PAULY

HOOVER INSTITUTION PRESS

STANFORD UNIVERSITY   STANFORD, CALIFORNIA

www.hoover.org

Hoover Institution Press Publication No. 580

Hoover Institution at Leland Stanford Junior University,
Stanford, California 94305-6010

First printing 2010
16   15   14   13   12   11   10   9   8   7   6   5   4   3   2   1

Manufactured in the United States of America

The paper used in this publication meets the minimum requirements of the American National Standard for Information Sciences—Permanence of Paper for Printed Library Materials, ANSI/NISO Z39.48-1992. ⊗

Cataloging-in-Publication Data is available from the Library of Congress.
ISBN-13: 978-0-8179-1044-0 (cloth. : alk. paper)
ISBN-13: 978-0-8179-1043-3 (e-book)

Contents

Foreword

Health care in the United States has made remarkable advances during the past sixty years. Dramatic improvements in diagnostic and therapeutic strategies, medical technologies, pharmaceuticals, and surgical procedures have extended the length and greatly improved the quality of life. Progress in the treatment of cardiovascular disease has reduced by more than 50 percent the U.S. death rate from heart attacks, accounting for nearly all the increases in the expected life span in the United States since 1950. Also, mainly as a result of the development of combination antiretroviral therapies for the treatment of AIDS, at least three million years of life have been cumulatively saved in the United States since 1989.

Despite such extraordinary progress, however, U.S. health care faces serious challenges. The problem is not so much that health care spending is high but that a significant portion of that spending fails to provide good value. As spending grows, an increasing number of people are priced out of the market for insurance. The fiscal burden of federal and state health care entitlement programs, such as Medicare and Medicaid, can no longer be sustained without either deep reductions in other public programs or sharply higher taxes. Diverting both public and private resources from more-productive uses has become a serious problem.

The debate over the direction of U.S. health care policy is occupying center stage in the domestic policy arena and will during the coming years. The promise of future medical advances stemming from the mapping of the human genome, nanotechnology, and other innovations is bright. But progress will require us to transcend the terms of the current debate, which are often expressed as the competing goals of universal insurance and cost control. The fundamental challenge is to devise public policies that enable more Americans to get better value for their health care dollar and foster appropriate innovation that extends and improves life. Key principles that guide policy formation should include the central role of individual choice and competitive markets in financing and delivering health services, individual responsibility for health behaviors and decisions, and appropriate guidelines for government intervention in health care markets.

The current core membership of the Hoover Institution's Working Group on Health Care Policy includes Scott W. Atlas, John F. Cogan, R. Glenn Hubbard, Daniel P. Kessler, Mark V. Pauly, and Charles E. Phelps.

JOHN RAISIAN
Tad and Dianne Taube Director,
Hoover Institution,
Stanford University
Stanford, California

Acknowledgments

I would like to thank those at the Hoover Institution, in particular John Cogan and Daniel Kessler, who supported and collaborated with me on this project. Special appreciation goes to Director John Raisian for creating the Working Group on Health Care Policy that provides a voice in the current policy debate on health care reform. I would also like to thank Henry Bergquist for excellent research assistance, Rob Liebenthal for useful discussions of the actuarial literature, and Bradley Herring for data on the distribution of the population by risk levels.

Health Reform without Side Effects

Making Markets Work for
Individual Health Insurance

MARK V. PAULY

Private health insurance in the United States protects most of the population against the risk of high medical care spending, but the extent of that protection has been declining for at least a decade. The reason for the decline appears to be no mystery: overall health insurance premiums for given coverage have been rising rapidly while consumer incomes have been near stagnant; consumers with little more to spend are increasingly reluctant to spend it on something with a rapidly growing price. But this simple story of prices growing relative to incomes is not quite right, and one piece of evidence arguing for a more nuanced approach is the well-known, widely varying susceptibility to this problem across the population. Most Americans are still getting good insurance protection for good medical care (at least in terms

1

of how they perceive their care), but for a sizeable fraction things are getting worse; not everything is broken, but some things for some people definitely are.

One of the flash points for this stressed system is the availability of insurance for consumers who do not find it easy to access the dominant form of private insurance. Most people are offered insurance related to their job, and most still take it. But increasingly large numbers of workers have jobs where coverage is not offered, or where the terms under which it is offered do not induce them to take it. It is the erosion of job-based coverage that is the main problem. There is an alternative to job-based insurance: consumers could buy health insurance in the same way they buy other kinds of insurance—voluntarily, as individual consumers, from private insurance firms. A small fraction (about 7% of the nonelderly population or 10% of those who have private insurance) do buy in this way.

However, the current individual insurance market is generally thought to not work well, less well, in most views, than even the misfiring employment-based market. In the individual market consumers tend to pay a lot for what they get, and, even with that, may worry about not being able to get and keep these overpriced products at all. Precisely because many of the uninsured appear to be permanent dropouts from the employment-based system, attention has turned to the development of an improved individual insurance alternative.

The current administration and Congress propose

changes and alternatives to this "nongroup" market, some quite dramatic and far-reaching. Are these new models the best, or are there other alternatives better matched to actual needs and with fewer adverse side effects? Can the current individual market serve as a foundation for reform, or must it be swept away, root and branch, and replaced with something entirely new? The current, most popular model of individual insurance reform proposes to revolutionize the way that market works, replacing the current market with a government-run insurance exchange offering a dominant public or consumer cooperative plan along with heavily regulated, privately managed alternatives. Consideration of its advantages and disadvantages may help in the choice between full replacement and modification.

I will begin with a discussion of the way in which individual insurance markets currently fit into the overall pattern of health insurance markets (considering both those who have and those who do not have insurance). I will then try to identify what is distinctive about current performance in that market relative to the alternatives: small-group private insurance, large-group private insurance, and public insurance. Finally, I will suggest improvements in the individual market that build on what currently works well, contrast these with alternative reforms, and offer a realistic assessment of how much improvement we can demand and expect.

My main conclusion is that, while there surely are some serious deficiencies in today's individual insurance market, the current criticisms are overly harsh, often based on anecdote and speculation, and ignore some important advantages in this market that should be preserved. I will also argue that the most frequently discussed alternative reforms reflect an excessively simplistic view of insurance markets that leads to policies likely to have serious adverse side effects, very likely to do more harm than good by driving out some of the beneficial features of the present market. I will argue that there are better approaches that take into account current strengths of the individual market and can yield much higher net benefits with much greater confidence.

Problem definition

Medical care is expensive because it is a prodigious consumer of high-value real resources, principally labor but also some capital and technology. In the long run, it can be made a little cheaper if consumers are willing to sacrifice some current features of care, but it cannot be made low cost. Its price can be temporarily lowered because some labor inputs (principally health professionals) have few equally attractive short-run alternatives: doctors' net incomes and nurses' wages can be squeezed for a while, although this only redistributes welfare and does not lower real resource cost and must be temporary. Health insurance premiums are high, and growing, because the medical costs they cover are high and growing. Health insurance and health care just cannot be made permanently "affordable" to low-income households except through subsidies. Someone has to pay for others, and someone has to decide how much to pay and for what.

However, medical care also provides high and growing benefits for our lives and those of our loved ones, and, on average and up to this time, the benefits appear to exceed the cost. So the nonpoor bulk of the population will still want care and would want it even if they have to pay the full high cost. To evaluate how well alternative ways of financing perform, we need therefore to begin by estimating how much care a household should have based on its own resources and then adding to that the contributions other citizens are willing to make if the household's own efforts fall short and it is thought to be in need.

How much care should a person have, and how should it best be paid for? We focus primarily on the nonpoor, because most of the population is not poor, but we deal as well with attempts to help the private individual market to work for low-income families. We begin with the premise that consumers should be well informed and that they should at least get the care they want and are willing to pay for on their own behalf. The pedantic economic planning model gives the same answer to this question as for all goods and services: the person should get care up to the point at which its additional benefit to that person equals its real resource cost given the person's health state and income. The person and the person's household should then pay for that care in a way that protects household wealth from the threat of high spending because of the uncertain occurrence of serious illness that is expensive to treat; there should be insurance.

These concepts of the ideal are abstract at this point, but they are more useful and more meaningful than some other suggested alternatives. People talk about the right to medical care, but they do not say how much is rightful or how it should be produced and paid for. Or they talk about "the right care of the right quality at the right time and at the right price" but do not tell us what "right" means. It surely does not mean what doctors would most prefer, or even what insured patients would most prefer (given in both cases that insurance is paying). Determining the benefit of more care to a given person requires knowing what the doctor knows (how sick the person is and what care provides what benefit), but this information must be combined with what the consumer-patient knows about the value placed on health outcomes relative to other uses of income and on side effects *and* costs (monetary and nonmonetary) of treatment.

Traditional health insurance usually gets in the way of making a good joint decision because it makes expensive services appear artificially cheap. There needs to be a trade-off between this inappropriate stimulus to high use and high cost (called "moral hazard" in the insurance literature), on the one hand, and financial risk protection on the other (Pauly 1968). With sufficient information, consumers of insurance can make all of these trade-offs, but getting the information can be challenging and costly. Still, it seems plausible that the bulk of people who are middle class and above choose enough coverage and enough care that others would not have great concern for (and be willing to pay much more for) their additional use of care or additional insurance benefits. If anything, among the middle class there is more overuse (benefit less than cost) than underuse (the reverse), and a solution to the problem of underuse for them is better and more persuasive information for those unaware of the benefits from care, not more insurance for all. As will be argued in more detail below, markets for care and markets for insurance for the nonpoor have no serious intrinsic impediments to good functioning, but they do require care and feeding and are easy to mess up.

For lower-income households in America (given moderate risk levels) and for high-risk households (given moderate income), this reasonable state of affairs does not apply. Generous subsidies for better care are needed for them. Fortunately, subsidized insurance can both provide financial protection and reverse moral hazard for community benefit, stimulating the use of care that others value more than the person can or does.

The majority of uninsured Americans are not poor, obtain their income from employment (including self-employment), but do not work in firms that offer them employment-based group insurance coverage. While reform could try to put many of these people into Medicaid or other public plan or (through an employer mandate) into employment-based insurance coverage, such changes would be large, awkward, and difficult. A more natural setting for covering the bulk of the uninsured is the setting already used by about 30% of people like them—the individual insurance market (Pauly, Percy, and Herring 1999). But this market is generally regarded (correctly, as we shall see, in its current form) as a relatively poor performer, both in terms of efficiency of administration and in terms of the efficiency-equity issues surrounding risk variation. In individual insurance, to put it bluntly, you pay a lot for what you get, and, if you are unfortunate enough to become a high risk, you pay even more or get even less. However, this bad reputation masks some real advantages to this market, even as it is, and, more importantly, inappropriately excludes this market from consideration for modifications that could reduce the bad features and enhance the good ones.

The lay of the land: How many people have what problems?

Not all parts of the private U.S. insurance market are yet in disarray. The market works well—at least as well as is possible, given the cost of health care—for very many people, but very poorly for others. We will use two measures of "works well." One is whether people end up obtaining insurance. The other is what they have to sacrifice to get insurance. The first indicator is measured by the proportion of those not receiving public coverage who have private coverage. The measure of the second indicator is more complex, since the alternative to paying nothing for health insurance is not usually getting good medical care for free; rather, it is being at risk for high out-of-pocket payments for constrained care of questionable quality or going without. The real cost of protecting yourself against the risk of uncertain medical spending is the difference between what you pay or would pay for health insurance and what you expect on average to get back as benefits. For a set of similar risks buying the same policy, this cost is the difference between total premiums paid and total benefits received; in insurance parlance this is called the "administrative loading" (or just "loading") on insurance. This measure of insurance price or cost is not perfect since it does not capture the offsetting benefit of getting more care than if one were uninsured, the offsetting cost of that care, and the nonmonetary cost of being limited in what care you can get and from whom by a managed care insurance plan. But it will do for a start. Economic theory and definitive empirical research tell us that the higher the loading, the less attractive is insurance, other things equal, and the more likely people are to choose to be

9

uninsured or not make strong efforts to become and stay insured. The punchline: the worst off a person or group can be is when they are often uninsured and would pay a high loading for insurance if they got it.

There are two primary determinants of who gets and keeps health insurance in the United States: decent income and employment at a large firm. The role of income is shown in Table 1. As indicated there, the likelihood of being uninsured for a person under 65 is only half as high if the person is in a household whose income is at or above 400% of the poverty line than if the person is poor or near poor, even with Medicaid as a public safety-net program for the poor.

Even so, uninsurance is not unknown among the middle class (the median U.S. household income is at about 325% of the poverty line), and a quarter of the uninsured (11.6 million out of 45 million) are above the 300% cutoff. (See also Yegian et al. 2000.) The table also shows that, at about 160% of poverty and above, most people somehow get private coverage. The implication is that, while income matters, there is more to coverage than just income or affordability.

Table 2 indicates the second major influence: firm size. The measure of size in this data is not ideal. We must look at "establishments" or places of employment, rather than firm size, because a large employer such as a fast-food chain may be composed of many small establishments. But since a large establishment cannot be part of a small firm, the measure still serves to indicate the effect of firm size, and the message is clear: even for

TABLE 1
Insurance Status of Individuals under 65 by Ratio of
Household Income to Federal Poverty Level (FPL)

Poverty Level		Uninsured	Government	Private	Total
<100%	n	11.4	17.0	5.7	34.1
	%	33.4%	49.8%	16.8%	100.0%
100–125%	n	3.6	4.5	3.1	11.2
	%	32.2%	40.5%	27.3%	100.0%
125–150%	n	3.7	3.8	4.0	11.5
	%	32.6%	33.1%	34.3%	100.0%
150–175%	n	2.8	2.9	4.7	10.5
	%	26.8%	28.1%	45.0%	100.0%
175–200%	n	3.0	2.4	5.5	10.9
	%	27.3%	21.9%	50.8%	100.0%
200–300%	n	8.8	7.0	27.9	43.7
	%	20.1%	16.0%	63.9%	100.0%
300–400%	n	4.6	3.8	28.3	36.7
	%	12.5%	10.4%	77.1%	100.0%
>400%	n	7.0	7.1	89.5	103.6
	%	6.8%	6.8%	86.4%	100.0%
Total	n	45.0	48.5	168.7	262.2

Source: Data from U.S. Census Bureau, Current Population Survey, March 2008
Supplement.
Note: Weighted (n in millions); individuals reporting both government and private
insurance are included in government insurance.

workers in relatively low-income households, insurance
is common if they work for a large employer, while well-
off workers at small firms may be uninsured.

I will discuss what are the "active ingredients" that
make insurance markets work well for large firms in

TABLE 2
Percentage of Uninsured Adults by Ratio of Household Income to
FPL and Establishment Size (households with a full-time worker)

Income as % of Poverty Line / Establishment Size	< 50 workers	≥ 50 workers
Below 300%	25.8%	13%
Above 300%	7.9%	2.3%

Source: Data from Centers for Disease Control and Prevention, National Center for Health Statistics, "National Health Interview Survey," 2008.
Note: Excludes unknown or other income categories.

more detail below, but for the present it is sufficient to note their relatively good performance in terms of both coverage and administrative cost. The few uninsured people who work full time in large firms are usually not eligible for coverage, often because they have just begun a job or are in a near-minimum-wage job, or, much more rarely, turned down offered coverage because they are not willing to pay the explicit employee premium. About 4% of the under-65 population offered employment-based insurance will not take insurance if they have to pay anything for it, no matter what. (For two-worker families, one worker will often enroll as a dependent on the spouse's plan.) The table further subdivides households with a large-firm worker by household income; there is a modest effect of income on the proportion with coverage but the proportion is above the national average regardless of household income.

There are two other employment-related categories: those who are employees at small firms and those who are not employees of any firm, either because they are self-employed or not working. Here the picture is quite different. In these categories, the number of uninsured is high, even among relatively high-income households. It is highest of all among people who do not at present have a group insurance option (although in principle anyone could try to get a job at a large firm); it is also high for middle-class people who work at small firms.

Can individual insurance help?

Those in households where no group insurance is offered (whether or not the person works as an employee) are "at risk" for purchasing individual insurance. Performance of this form of insurance is not impressive; in this case, insurance reaches only about 25% of the population. But many of those who work as employees could have taken jobs at firms offering coverage. A sub-population with no alternative but individual insurance would be those who are self-employed or not employed; here the proportion with coverage is still low, at about a third (Marquis et al. 2006).

The proportion of the population with private insurance has been trending downward, to some extent offset (and perhaps caused) by expansion of public coverage, especially through Medicaid and the State Children's Health Insurance Program (SCHIP). The fall in private coverage has not generally occurred among people in households with a worker at a large firm, in part because such firms continue to offer coverage and in part because household incomes for workers at large firms are higher and therefore less subject to crowd-out from public plans. Moreover, although the data is somewhat soft, it appears that the erosion in coverage for workers at small firms does not largely result from firms dropping existing coverage, but rather from firms that do not offer coverage replacing firms that did. There has also been some tightening of eligibility so that more workers in firms that offer coverage do not qualify.

Table 3 provides some rough data on the components of administrative cost for insurance bought as group coverage or as individual coverage. The loading is higher the smaller the group, and it is also more vari-

TABLE 3
Components of Insurer Administrative Costs
(as percentage of claims)

Group Size	Commissions	General Admin.	Profit (net)	Taxes[a]	Claims	Total
Individual	N/A	N/A	N/A	N/A	N/A	40–100%
1–20	8%	11%	7%	3%	5%	34%
100–500	1.6%	4%	4%	2.3%	4%	16%
10,000 +	0.1%	0.7%	0%	2.1%	3%	4–6%

Source: Author's calculations based on data from the Congressional Research Service (2000).
[a]Avoided if firm self-insures

able. This pattern and its rationale will be discussed in more detail below, but the main message is clear: the administrative loading, and therefore the true price of insurance, is much higher for individual than large-group insurance. This table differs from the original calculations (created by the Hay Group in 1999) in reducing the estimated charge for claims processing to a more uniform percentage; it also makes an estimate for individual coverage based on extrapolating the very small group numbers and using other evidence in the informal literature.

The time trend in the loading percentage has been modestly upward across the board; the average loading in private insurance has probably increased by 1 to 1.5% of premiums over the last 20 years. This is largely due to the spread of managed care, which is somewhat more costly to administer (per dollar of benefits or premium) than was old-style insurance, which just paid claims but did not select panels of providers, preapprove coverage, or attempt to manage care. This growth in cost seems to be fairly uniform by group size on average, although anecdotes of substantial increases in premiums are much more common in the small-group and individual markets; there is more dispersion in premiums in such markets.

The extent of competition among private insurers measured by firm market shares (in states or cities) has never been very high. In most areas, the Blue Cross and Blue Shield plans have dominated for many decades, often with market shares in the 80–90% range. The share of the largest non-Blue for-profit plan has never been greater than 25%. There have been some exceptions and some changes to these generalizations. In California and New York the Blue plans were never as dominant, and both private for-profit insurers and independent managed care plans were important. There has been consolidation and change during the past decade; the independent HMOs were bought up or disappeared, some of the Blue plans converted to being investor owned, and the separate Blue plans with different geographic territories merged. Data are soft here as well because some consumers have policies from more than one firm and because self-insured employers really do not buy insurance from any insurance firm, even if they use an insurance company to process claims or organize panels to supply medical services.

The Blues still dominate, with about 100 million out of about 170 million total privately insured. Accounting for the Blue plans that are non-investor-owned, the market splits about 50–50 between for-profit and nonprofit or mutual (consumer cooperative) firms. Historically, the Blue plans were typically even more important than other insurers in the individual market, although United Health Care now has a substantial individual presence due to its acquisition of Golden Rule Insurance, and the investor-owned (but Blue) Wellpoint firm is active in the individual market as well (though individual insureds are only about 7% of the total population for which it administers insurance). Only concentration, not ownership form, appears to affect competition, and there is some evidence that high concentration in managed care does lead to monopoly behavior in the HMO market (though not necessarily in the overall health insurance market) (Pauly et al. 2002). Profit levels do not yet signal generally high market power, even when the number of insurers selling in a market is small; net income of private insurers was negative or very low in the later 1990s, and has recovered, but profits as a proportion of premiums rarely exceed 5%. The local markets in which one insurer is dominant are always dominated by a Blue firm, which is usually nonprofit and subject to greater state scrutiny than commercial insurers.

There is, however, more competition among insurers than simple market-share measures would suggest. For one thing, most large groups self-insure, purchasing administrative services only (or some reinsurance) from the private insurers. These large buyers would not tolerate prices (for coverage or administrative services) that yield high insurer profits because they can turn both to administrative-services-only firms (such as benefits consultants) and plans in other states to provide those services. Smaller employers and individuals are more vulnerable. Even here, however, there is potential entry into the pure insurance business should any existing insurer try to exercise serious market power. The main possible source of power is not insurance per se (performing the function of pooling risk); when there is

17

market power it comes from a dominant insurer's provider network and/or management tools, which new entrants may find hard to duplicate. Still, while consolidation in the industry is troubling, such changes do not appear to be major factors in increasing premiums or reducing the proportion of the population with coverage.

There does not appear to be comprehensive data on the profitability of individual insurance. For-profit health insurers as a whole earned a pretax return on equity in 2008 of about 8% to 11%, a moderate rate by the standard of other industries. They earned a low rate (at 2% to 4%) as a proportion of revenues; cutting profits in half would produce a barely noticeable reduction in premiums. The return on equity of Golden Rule Insurance, the largest company specializing in individual insurance before it was acquired by United Health Care, was about 7% in 2000. This line of insurance does not appear to be so profitable that it is attracting entry or growth; the recent moderate expansion by Wellpoint was offset by the exit in 2002 of Mutual of Omaha, which had been a major player. Profits for this type of insurance are not consistently out of line or above average relative to competitive returns elsewhere in the economy. Individual insurer profits are in the billions of dollars but are a tiny fraction of the industry's total revenue and costs, which are in the hundreds of billions. More recent (but incomplete) data found the average margin as a percentage of premiums for individual insurance to be about 2% or less in 2008, though it showed a loss for small-group insurance (Austin and Hungerford 2009).

Coverage for high risks

One of the main criticisms of individual insurance, and one of the main motivations for dramatic increases in regulation, has to do with the belief that the individual markets treat poorly people of substantially greater risk than average. As we will show, this is true to a considerable extent, but group insurance does an equally poor (or worse) job of protecting high risks, especially those who work for small firms. But we first want to make a key point about relative importance: *compared to the number of people under 65 who are average or normal risks, the fraction who are high risks is very small.*

In some ways, the point should be so obvious as to be undeserving of italics: the country cannot be some kind of perverse Lake Wobegon in which everyone is an above-average risk. In fact, as well shall see, the shape of the distribution of risk levels is skewed to the right, meaning that most people are below-average risks and the average is driven up by only relatively few high risks. This point is important because common sense would suggest that if the problem of high risks is relatively rare, it would not generally be necessary to make drastic changes in markets for the great majority of the popula-

19

tion; instead, specialized interventions targeted at the small minority of high risks (with associated modest impacts on the rest of the population) would be more efficient, more transparent, and more feasible. (As we will see, the small fraction of high risks is a different phenomenon from the rarity of a high-cost illness for a person of average risk; in the latter case, insurance is designed to deal with the rare event that has yet to happen but could occur.)

There is no definitive measure of the proportion of the under-65 population not covered by Medicaid or Medicare (as disabled or with kidney failure) who are high risk. Estimates of the proportion who are "uninsurable" are as low as less than 1% (Frakt, Pizer, and Vrobel 2004), but I believe a reasonable number is the proportion with high-cost chronic conditions, which is about 4% of this population (Pauly and Herring 1999). (This is the average proportion with expected expenses due to chronic conditions that are more than twice the average, controlling for demographic characteristics; the proportion with expenses more than three times the average is 2%.) An implication of this small proportion is that the problem of a person becoming a high risk just about the time individual insurance is initiated should be even more rare, so the problem of preexisting-condition exclusions must affect only a tiny fraction of the population (7% with individual insurance times 4% high risk times the probability of becoming high risk just when the individual sets out to buy insurance has to result in a tiny number). There will still be "many thousands" of people with such problems, so something should be done, but they make up such a small share of the total that wholesale changes hardly seem needed.

Risk in health policy analysis has many meanings (Pauly 2007), but the one to be discussed here is the risk of medical care spending (that will potentially be covered wholly or in part by insurance). *Risk* in this sense means expected or predicted medical spending; a person will be said to be a high risk if, based on current characteristics (such as age, ethnicity, health condition), the person would be expected to have expenses much above average. This meaning is to be contrasted with the use of the term *risk* in the phrase "risk pooling." In risk pooling properly defined, risk is discussed in the context of a population with the same expected medical spending whose actual spending will vary substantially depending on the random pattern of events. What is pooled is the unknown that is yet to happen, not the consequences of known events that have already occurred. (Risk pooling will be discussed in more detail later.)

One common characterization of medical care spending is that it follows the "80–20 rule": in any year, 80% of spending is associated with 20% of the population that gets really sick; the other 4 out of 5 people are reasonably healthy and so spend less on average and in total. Sometimes it is said that this fact alone shows that there will be a potential problem with treatment of high risks. For example, Charlie Baker of Partners Health (2009) observed, "20% of the population incurs 80% of the costs, and vice versa. That's called risk pooling, and it's why Massachusetts (and Hillary Clinton during her presidential campaign) called for mandating health insurance coverage as part of the state's reform efforts." While Baker's discussion of the "rule" is accurate, his conclusion about the need for mandating is not necessarily correct: even if people were all of the same risk, the uncertain incidence of illness would result in some spending much more than others, but all might well voluntarily purchase insurance to spread this risk. Indeed, the whole basis of insurance is that people of the same risk level at the beginning of a period can expect to realize quite different loss levels over the period; insurance converts this lottery on bad outcomes into a uniform premium that all may pay and therefore end up no worse off financially regardless of what actually happens.

What is crucial to the policy discussion instead is the distribution of risk, and that in turn depends on the distribution of characteristics that predict high spending, a distribution that, as it turns out, does not fit the 80–20 rule. There are more truly low risks and fewer truly high risks than would be indicated by the rule, especially at the extremes of the distribution of losses. However, it remains true that risk is unevenly distributed and distributed in the skewed fashion implied by the rule.

Community rating: the worst possible way to do a good thing

There is a strong case (to be treated in more detail later) that can be made against simple annual risk-rating of health insurance and its anticipated effects on high risks. The problem is this: annual risk rating would expose people to risk. The risk they confront is called "reclassification risk" and represents the possibility that unexpected onset of a chronic condition may cause a person's future health insurance premiums (under simple annual risk rating) to take a big jump. Not only may this make insurance unaffordable for lower-income high risks, but it also makes those who might become high risks at all income levels more miserable than they need to be.

In the recent policy proposals from the Obama administration and the Democratic Congress, the solution to this problem that is most obvious but has the worst side effects is the one that has been virtually the sole topic of discussion: regulate premiums by requiring insurers to charge buyers with different expected expenses under a given policy the same premium—so-called "community rating"—and close any loopholes by forbidding insurers from limiting coverage for preexisting conditions at this premium. There has been almost no dissent expressing the general undesirability of this approach.

There are strong arguments against community rating in the insurance literature (Pauly 1970). It is therefore somewhat surprising (if not disappointing) that this old clunker has such a powerful grip on policymakers. Here is the simple critical argument in the literature. Assume that competitive insurers can perfectly distinguish risk and so set premiums based on risk (so there is no reason to expect adverse selection or cream-skimming). Higher-than-average premiums for people who become higher-than-average risks have some undesirable effects (just mentioned), so it is good public policy to assume that those higher premiums are cushioned in some way. There may also be a social equity motivation for cushioning the financial status of those who become high risks, even those with moderate incomes. A good way to do so is to allow insurers to charge risk-rated buyers higher premiums but then to subsidize those premiums for those high-risk buyers who are thought to be deserving of help—either because they unexpectedly became high risk (risk reclassification) or because there is societal concern about their ability to buy health insurance (unaffordability). The money for this subsidy should be raised by the most efficient and equitable tax available, usually thought to be the general income tax, although a value added tax would possibly be superior. Other than some administrative complexities concerned with identifying the targets for subsidy and making sure the subsidy itself does not distort the amount of insurance bought, this simple policy solves the problem.

In the ideal arrangement, no price regulation is needed; insurers should be able to charge more for high risks. Community rating is a much inferior solution strategy. The most serious unintended adverse consequence is that, if it is implemented in otherwise competitive insurance markets without targeted subsidies, insurers required to underprice (relative to expected benefits cost plus loading) for higher risks must overprice policies sold to lower risks in order to cover their total cost. The consequence of this price distortion is that lower risks will drop or fail to buy coverage. There is substantial evidence that this is what happens, and to such an extent that community rating actually causes more people in total to be uninsured, even as it modestly reduces the number of uninsured high risks. Herring and Pauly (2007) found that rate regulation slightly increased the relative likelihood that a high risk would get individual coverage (from 0.96 of the low risk likelihood to equal likelihood) but that the increase in low-risk premiums would increase the overall uninsured population, as more low risks were driven out than high risks were brought in. Case studies of the initiation and functioning of community rating in different states have failed to find evidence that it helps with the problem of the uninsured, or even that it consistently helps significant numbers of high-risk uninsured, compared to no rate regulation (Swartz and Garnick 2000; Chollett and Kirk 1998). Often it results in a meltdown of the entire individual market as companies withdraw from that business. It does provide more employment for insurance regulators.

One might still prefer community rating to doing nothing, if one attaches high enough value to covering the high risks and low enough or no negative value to increasing the number of low-risk uninsured, but the point of insurance theory is that there is a better alternative to doing nothing that does not have this side effect. Formally, community rating can be thought of as financing a subsidy to insurance for higher risks (there being potential social value to the subsidy) through an excise tax on insurance sold to lower risks. The economics just reviewed tells us to avoid specific excise taxes in favor of more general taxes. The alternative subsidy/financing model outlined above does just that; there is no reason to think that higher income taxes would appreciably affect the insurance purchasing plans of anyone, regardless of risk level. From the viewpoint of economic efficiency, subsidizing high risks is often desirable, but paying for that subsidy by taxing low risks never is. Nor is there an obvious equity reason why low risks should pay. The reason for the political appeal of this policy is that the tax on low risks is not counted as a tax, does not show up on any budget, and is opaque for all, even to low risks who are likely to blame the insurers, not the regulators, for their high premiums.

The primary rationale for community rating, it is important to note, is not adverse selection that arises from intrinsically better knowledge of risk by buyers than sellers. Rather, the targeted policy problem is risk rating where the insurer actually has figured out who is higher-than-average risk and is proposing to charge that person more than average and likewise to charge less than average to low risks. Community rating will then *cause* adverse selection (and its supply-side mirror image, cream-skimming) when it did not have to exist. There are theoretical reasons to consider community rating as a solution to the problem of true adverse selection, but the rarity of this case combined with the availability of alternative ways to ensure that low risks remain in the market (such as subsidies or mandates) diminish the importance of this argument.[1]

Certainly one of the most ironic recent studies is a Commonwealth Fund study that asserts that reform, with community rating as its centerpiece, will help young people and lower risks to get coverage. It notes proposals for state regulations requiring insurers to per-

---

1. Even here, a pooled policy charging the same premiums and selling the same coverage to high and low risks may temporarily emerge, either because of community-rating rules or because it is preferred by low risks to very skimpy though cheap coverage. But then insurers and low risks will realize that there is another policy, at a premium based on the low-risk rate though somewhat less generous than the pooled one, that the low risks will prefer but the high risks will not—so the market cannot be stable. But for-bidding this policy will make the low risks worse off. Mandatory community-rated basic coverage can sometimes improve effi-ciency if people at different risk levels are permitted to supplement in different ways.

mit parents to keep dependents on their policies after age 23 (at higher premiums) without noting the absence of evidence that such provisions make a difference. The most striking omission is the failure to note that major reform proposals would have the effect (through community rating that limits appropriate risk adjustments for age) of dramatically raising premiums for young people. Some of the reform proposals allow somewhat lower premiums for young people, but the reduction is much less than what would be consistent with their lower risk. Even the subsidies offered for some young people are unlikely to change their (correct) perception that overpriced insurance is a less attractive buy, one that rational young people will reject. There is no better way to drive more healthy young people out of the individual market than to implement proposed insurance reforms.

In addition to the flaw of distorted prices, the regulatory process associated with community rating generates a host of other problems. It provides incentives to insurers to avoid or underserve high risks (when formerly at risk-rated premiums, selling insurance to high risks would be profitable). Rules need to be put in place to risk-adjust the revenues insurers will collect, adjustments that are bound to be imperfect. So then there must be heavy regulations to close off all avenues by which lower risks and insurers conspire together to avoid the cross subsidy: policy design, marketing, innovation, prevention programs, and provider networks all must be controlled. Finally, the doors are thrown open for political and special interests to lobby: public health types against patient cost-sharing, managed care opponents against aggressive plans, and politicians for whichever provider or insurer group wants to make sure that they are part of the preferred plan, all in the name of keeping out plans that might appeal to low risks. Imagination will be stifled, the uninsured will increase, and political rent-seeking will be rampant.

So as the discussion of health reform shifts to that of health *insurance* reform, it is important to note that the centerpiece of congressional legislation—federal community-rating regulation—will itself increase the general incentives for the group already most at risk of being uninsured, the good risks, to become even more likely to be uninsured. Far from being an inevitable consequence of health reform intended to assure coverage of high risks, this adverse effect of community rating can be avoided by choosing a different way to reform the individual market.

What's wrong with individual insurance?

Individual insurance, with or without community rating, has its serious problems, too. The primary problem with individual insurance concerns its pricing. Its high administrative cost makes its average price high, and there is substantial variation in prices for the same product across sellers. That is, regardless of risk level, individual premiums are high and variable relative to the benefits received. There appears to be substantial variation in the ratio of premiums to expected benefits across different insurers' individual products, as well as variation across risk groups. The result is that, no matter what your age and risk level, if you enter the individual market you will face the unlovely prospect of high and varying prices for essentially the same product, along with a great variety of products. Getting a reasonably good deal is not going to be easy and (depending on how you define "good") may not be possible. As a result, some transactions occur at high prices, and all transactions occur at premiums that are considerably higher than benefits received. A potential partial solution to this problem is to use an insurance broker to help find a good price for a good product, but brokers add commissions of their own.

There is no definitive data on administrative costs (or, as already noted, profit margins) across the set of all individual insurance options in a local market.[2] From the information we have, it appears that the medical loss ratio—the proportion of premiums actually paid out each year as benefits—is about 65% to 75% in the indi-

---

2. We can and will make some rough calculations about the observed aggregate average ratio of premiums to benefits, but, because insurance markets are local, this is not necessarily a good measure of what a given person will face.

vidual market. What does not go for benefits goes to pay administrative costs (the "loading") and profits.

Good comprehensive data on the components of individual insurance loading is even harder to find, but it does appear that the cost of processing claims in individual markets is comparable to that in group insurance markets, at about 4% to 6% of premiums. This should be no surprise, because insurers who sell individual products usually also sell group and network products and use the same claims-payment mechanisms for all their business. And, as already noted, profits (for the minority of for-profit individual insurers) or "surplus revenues" (for the nonprofits) appear to be a small fraction of premiums.

It is the other two main categories of expense—selling costs and general administration—that are much higher in the individual market than in other public or private group markets. The agent or entity that persuades someone to buy this high-priced insurance will have to be paid.

Although an agent who sells a given policy to a large group will get a higher commission than if the same policy were sold to an individual, the commission rises much less than proportionately—so the commission per new person insured is much higher for the single-person sale than for the multiple-person one. General administration costs are also higher per person. These costs go for billing and collection of premiums and for answering policyholders' questions. There are also economies of scale in billing: compared to individuals, larger groups spread billing costs over more people, and they also typically pay on time with less (costly) nagging from the seller and fewer confused inquiries from the buyer. Surprisingly, most states add insult to injury by taxing health insurance premiums under their jurisdiction (as they tax premiums for other kinds of insurance), generally at about 2% of premiums, though the tax goes as high as 10% of premiums in New York. State taxes on insurances are a major source of revenue, sometimes the third largest component (behind income and sales taxes). While 2% sounds relatively modest, it would represent a 13% increase in the net cost of coverage (premiums minus benefits) for a policy with a typical 15% loading. State government revenue-raising adds almost as much to individual insurance premiums as do the profits that private and public insurers (averaged over for-profit and nonprofit) receive. It is ironic that states ask for federal funding for new programs to cover uninsured children and high risks when they are imposing taxes that cause more people to be uninsured.

What is perhaps surprising is that the direct cost of underwriting—the process by which an application for coverage is reviewed, accepted, or rejected, and if accepted, quoted a premium that will be related to some extent to risk—is actually a trivial fraction, surely less than 0.5%, of administrative costs. And, as we shall see, for the person who buys a policy and then renews that coverage for subsequent time periods, underwriting is done only once—so any cost gets spread over time.

The other potentially surprising omission is that there need not be any contribution to higher charges related to supposed lower "risk spreading" in the individual market. The combination of a one-year time frame for insurance along with the bundling of thousands of individual applicants into a single risk portfolio means that, even in individual markets, the potentially wide variation in what can happen to any one person cancels out across thousands, and so should generate no additional charge for risk bearing per se. To be sure, actuaries in their calculations of suggested premiums will sometimes add a charge for risk in recognition of the risk-pooling benefit provided to individual consumers, but since that benefit has no cost to the insurer, that charge will not be supported in a competitive market. And, as noted above, profits on individual insurance appear to be close to the competitive level.

There are other potential risks of the individual market—for example, less reliable data on the risk of any one buyer and the attendant possibility of the "winner's curse" in which buyers gravitate toward the most (overly) optimistic seller. But there is no quantification of this risk—it is similar to the risk in any business where prices are set too low compared to what costs turn out to be—and in any case it should be pooled in equity markets. There may be an actuarial fudge factor applied to estimated claims to account for persistent underestimation of risk for people who choose to buy, but this does not add to cost; it just corrects the underestimate. In the more reliable group data, this "charge" would have been included in an accurate estimate of annual benefits cost; it is no higher a cost in individual markets than in other insurance markets. More generally, there should be no risk charge for an estimate that takes the same value year in and year out.

It is sometimes argued that people with higher-than-average expected expenses will not have their "risk" (which is not a true risk, of something yet to happen) pooled with lower-than-average risks in individual markets, in line with the supposed risk-pooling function of insurance markets (Pauly 2007). But if higher risks fare less well in individual markets—something which, as we shall see, is not always necessarily the case—lower risks will fare better. So, on balance, individual markets do not harm the average risk. People in individual markets cannot all be higher risks by the law of averages. The median risk, who is actually below the mean, will not pay more for individual insurance for this reason. Voluntary insurance markets are not intended to pool the risk of things that have already happened. If group insurance markets really do anything fundamentally different about variation in individuals' risk from individual insurance markets (something that is far from certain), they do not "risk pool"; if they do anything, they "risk average" or "risk-based transfer."

A clear way to see the difference between risk averaging and risk pooling is to consider situations in which high risks and low risks buy comprehensive insurance coverage and pay a community rate. Because coverage is complete, consumers bear no risk, and only pay a premium they know with certainty. But now let community rating be replaced with risk rating. If coverage remains the same, consumers still bear no risk of out-of-pocket payments depending on whether or not they get sick. And they still can expect to pay premia they know with certainty. The only distinction is that the certain premiums are different from before, higher for higher risks and lower for lower risks. Compared to risk rating, community rating does not lower aggregate risk; it only makes transfers from low to high risks.

The administrative loading in individual insurance is greater than in employment-based group insurance (employer resources handle insurance issues, so some group-insurance costs are transferred from insurer to employer). However, the individual insurance loading approximates that in most other insurances that people buy as individuals: homeowners' insurance, automobile collision coverage, and tenants' insurance (Kunreuther, Pauly, and McMorrow, forthcoming). Term life insurance and auto liability insurance appear modestly less costly to administer, but, in the former case, purchases once made are usually repeated automatically (and at little administrative cost) year after year, and, in the latter case, the resources used to determine the value of claims are generated by the legal system and incorporated into the benefit payouts, and so are not counted as insurer costs. Individual health insurance is expensive because it costs a lot to administer.

There are potential ways to improve administrative efficiency in the individual market, but high administrative costs do not show that there is intrinsic inefficiency (or, apparently, higher-than-competitive profits) in this market, given the product it offers, the production process for that product, and the channel used to offer it.

The wide pricing variation for similar products already noted does, however, seem to be a defect. Wide variation in prices apparently does not translate into high insurer profits across the board; this is not a market where all confused buyers are ripped off. As we will note below, there is evidence that the bulk of buyers eventually do find their way to reasonably good deals—more so the more money there is at stake. The real inefficiency here is the direct and indirect cost of buyer search, along with the riskiness inherent in the whole process. The advent of online selling of individual insurance may have helped somewhat in recent years.

Still, there is a strong element of arbitrary and capricious disarray in the individual market that has given it an appropriately tainted reputation. Add the occasional tale of a scandalous company pulling fast ones on its customers, hiding in fine print, and reneging on implicit promises, and it is no surprise that this market does not have defenders even among those who will want to use it. For example, Douglas Holtz-Eakin, then advisor to

Senator John McCain, said that "the current individual market is not a good place to live" (2007). He then went on to overstate things a bit: "There is nothing in the individual market that everybody should embrace and love." I disagree. I will argue that there are some things in this market that could be embraced (though not necessarily loved). The generally jaundiced view health policy analysts of all stripes have of the individual market is not undeserved, but there are some advantages to that market which reform should cultivate rather than discard.

What is good about the individual market?

Some of the advantages of the individual market are mirror images of the disadvantages associated with its administrative cost and pricing variation. One advantage is that the individual person has a wide choice of what policy to take rather than being limited to the policy or set of policies offered in a group. In a sense, the higher administrative cost of individual insurance is in part the cost of variety. Variety will be most valued by people whose choice would have been different from what the group would have chosen, so this is an advantage that will have varying values across people; the individual market is more valuable to eccentrics than to conformists. An aspect which should be valuable to all is that the individual controls the choice, rather than an employer, a union, or a benefits department. In individual markets the person does not have to worry that some other agent, such as the employer or team of benefits consultants, will decide to change the policy or even change the pricing of the policy.

In the group health insurance market, you get it cheap, but you get what someone else wants. Employers often are confused by their health benefits and make arbitrary decisions to cut benefits even when their employees would prefer more generous benefits and would be prepared to take lower raises to pay for them. In the individual market, the only relevant confusion is that of the buyer—and the buyer has the option of obtaining reasonably good advice from brokers or financial counselors, though at a price. This does not, I must hasten to add, mean that the person would not prefer the group market. Even if consumers do not get exactly what they want, they may still be happy if it is a lot lower in cost and not too different from what they most like.

The variety of choices in the individual market is to some extent limited by what is available in the area—in Philadelphia I cannot choose a group- or staff-model HMO, such as Kaiser—but the restriction is much less than in group settings. The number of choices offered to people in employment-based settings tends to shrink as firm size shrinks. Very many people who get group insurance from small employers have no choice at all. So the people working for small firms—who are paying loadings not very much lower than in individual insurance—actually can buy much more choice with relatively little money by moving to the individual market. They do not get much reward for going along with the group. So why not embrace the individual market, in principle, at least? As we will see, it will also offer important risk protection that small-group coverage is lacking.

There is an important policy divide here. If you think that almost everyone (properly informed) would truly want about the same kind of health insurance—similar in both extent of out-of-pocket payment and strictness of managed care policies—then the case for the individual market, or any market, is greatly weakened. Even an imperfect government should be able to figure out what almost everyone wants if they all want the same thing, and provide it at low administrative cost. The case for markets rests on the hypothesis of—and the evidence for—variation in what people want from their health insurance. The current pattern in which workers, given a choice, do sort themselves across a range of policies from generous to frugal, and from permissive to restrictive, does strongly suggest that, at least in the United States, there is substantial preference variation. (There is also evidence of variation from some other countries, such as Switzerland; despite what politicians favoring solidarity may say, people are different.) Similar variation across the Medicare population—in the amount and type of Medigap chosen, or in the form of the

Part D plan, likewise suggests different preferences. Markets, not government, are best at providing different things to different people.

Another advantage of the individual market is portability. As the person changes jobs, takes off from work for a period of time, or moves to self-employment, he or she can retain the same coverage at the same price. With group insurance, even after the passage of the Health Insurance Portability and Accountability Act (HIPAA), a person who changes jobs often must change benefits—and learn a whole new system. There is also the possibility that the person will not take a job at which he could be more productive because he does not want to change benefits. This is in part the notorious "job lock," which the Clinton plan for using local health insurance purchasing cooperatives was supposed to alleviate, but it would not be a problem in the first place if workers had their insurance as individuals.

These first two advantages of today's individual insurance are fairly obvious. The third advantage is less obvious. One of the threats to a family's economic as well as physical health is the unexpected onset of a high-cost chronic condition. Even with good insurance to cushion the often high explicit costs associated with first symptoms and diagnosis, the person faces the future prospect (until going on Medicare at age 65 or becoming so incapacitated as to be disabled) of being a high risk, someone insurers reasonably expect to incur above-average medical costs under any given policy. In an ordinary insurance market, a high-cost insurance product, without a subsidy, would have to sell at a high price, and so consumers rightly fear the compounding of their bad luck as poor future health is accompanied by very high future insurance premiums, incomplete coverage, or no coverage at all.

This dire prospect is a real threat for all healthy Americans, and anecdotes abound of the misery experienced even by middle-class people (uninsured or with group insurance they lose) who unexpectedly become high risks. The great bulk of individual insurance, even without further reforms, offers good protection against this fate for people who were able and willing to anticipate its possibility and buy individual insurance before they got sick. In particular, except for bridging insurance explicitly labeled as temporary, all individual insurance now must contain a provision for "guaranteed renewability at class average rates."[3] That is, the insurer promises to renew coverage each year if the person pays the new premiums, for everyone who becomes a high risk since initially buying, and it promises that the new premiums will not be increased selectively because of the onset of this condition (or for any other reason). Premiums can be increased, but they must be increased the same for all in a given rating or risk class. This feature

---

3. President Obama's comment that his health plan will prevent insurers from "raising your premiums or canceling your coverage" thus does not differ from the individual market.

solves the problem of "reclassification risk" (Pauly, Kunreuther, and Hirth 1995; Cochrane 1995).

This provision was present in most individual insurance policies for many years (since it avoids the cost of "re-underwriting") before any state or federal regulation and is now required as part of state regulation by the federal HIPAA law (Patel and Pauly 2002). While the data for the pre-HIPAA period are imprecise and combine health and disability insurance, it is estimated that 80% of individual insurance contained guaranteed renewability provisions even before the federal law and its effect on state laws (Pauly, Percy, and Herring 1999). Thus, arguments in the health reform debate that, after reform, insurers will not be allowed to "drop you if you get sick" are largely beside the point for individual insurance since federal regulation already forbids such behavior.[4]

That guaranteed renewability is a real commitment from an insurer's point of view is supported by its treatment in the actuarial literature. That literature emphasizes that the premiums for health insurance with guaranteed renewability have to be larger than those just needed to cover current-period expected expenses in order to accumulate funds to pay higher costs of insureds who become high risks in future periods. Generally, the actuary will set up a contract reserve to cover

---

4. Another potential benefit from guaranteed renewability is that it gives strong incentives to the insurer to keep their insureds healthy and thus avoid costly chronic conditions.

this commitment. Actuaries note that arbitrary actions which would force out high risks would deprive them of their "premium equity" in the policy.

There is a debate in the actuarial literature about the possibility that insurers should or could act in ways that undermine the guarantee (Bluhm 2006, 2007). The controversy over durational rating, where the time since the contract was first written defines a rating class (and often leads to an increase in premiums for contracts of longer duration), is about whether such rating is consistent with guaranteed renewability or undermines it. The controversy is not settled, but actuaries do generally advise that insurers limit themselves to cancellations or rate increases strictly on a class underwriting basis, so at least part of the guaranteed renewability promise not to single out high risks for high premiums is preserved. Actuaries apparently are divided on whether insurers could or should use more strategic activities to shed higher risks.

While there are some ways an insurer willing to tarnish its reputation or abandon its individual business can avoid the limits imposed by guaranteed renewability provisions, this behavior appears to be uncommon. The best evidence that this good behavior actually occurs on a large scale is from data on the relationship between premiums actually paid for individual insurance and the risk level of the person buying it (Herring and Pauly 2007). Analysis of this data indicates that there is a great deal of risk pooling—up to 60% for demographic variation and up to 85% for chronic conditions, given a person's age, gender, family situation, and location. That is, only about 15% of the higher cost of a chronic condition actually shows up in higher premiums paid by people with such conditions in the individual market; much of the variation in risk is not reflected in premiums. So, not only is individual insurance portable, on the same terms and at the same premiums, across jobs, it is also similarly portable across health conditions. The net effect of such a provision is that higher risks in the overall individual market are almost as likely as lower risks to end up with individual coverage—even without subsidies and even without rate regulation. Additional work by Bundorf, Herring, and Pauly (forthcoming) that looked only at employed people and their families found that high risks were actually *more* likely to have coverage.

There is also other convincing and consistent empirical evidence. Individual insurance premiums are front-loaded, as the theory predicts; they are higher relative to expected expenses for young buyers than for older ones (Pauly and Herring 1999). And the age profile of individual premiums actually paid is consistent with the path theory would suggest (Pauly and Herring 2006). Despite anecdotes and worries about insurers reneging, aggregate data on the individual insurance market looks much as it should if guaranteed renewability is working.

A key point is that group insurance does *not* at present have the same kind of protection against risk reclassification as does individual insurance. As long as the person stays in the group (keeps the job), both regulation and customary practice do prevent explicit group premiums from varying with risk. However, there are no insurance regulations that prevent money wages from reflecting risk to some extent, and there is some evidence that wages are lower for those with high-risk conditions, such as obesity, or who are older (Sheiner 1999; Pauly and Herring 1999). Even more to the point, the high-risk person who leaves employment at the insured job loses protection against re-underwriting and risk rating. Indeed, research shows that workers in poor health who were covered by small-group insurance in one year are nearly twice as likely to be uninsured in the next year than were workers with similar health status who had individual coverage (Pauly and Lieberthal 2008). Ironically, when a high-risk person loses group coverage and then seeks individual insurance only to be treated as a high risk, it is the individual insurer who is often excoriated for proposing to charge a high-risk rated and underwritten premium, even though it was group insurance, with no guarantee of renewability, that lured the person to buy insurance that then plunged him into this predicament. Exploring the possibility of adding guaranteed renewability to group insurance *for the individual worker*, not for the employer or group, seems highly desirable. However, employers who offer health benefits for the purpose of attracting and retaining good workers may not be so eager to have such insurance easily portable across jobs.

How not to critique the individual health insurance market

Analysts at the Commonwealth Fund recently published a report that concluded that "the individual market in its current form does not provide a viable alternative to employer-based group coverage" (2009, 2). Even though the study does correctly point out some problems with the individual market, the bulk of its analysis is irrelevant, and its conclusion is incorrect. Reform is needed in the individual market, but this kind of work is not helpful.

The analysis is based on a 2007 survey funded by the foundation that surveyed people who were not currently enrolled in group insurance. The survey simply asked people if they ever "tried to buy" individual insurance, without defining "try" or asking about the circumstances. In the sample of about 1,600 respondents, a third said they "tried to buy" individual insurance and a total of 130 did end up with individual coverage. What happened to those who "tried" at some point but did not buy individual coverage is not shown. Some may have remained uninsured, but surely many others obtained group coverage or went on Medicaid.

The reasons of high price and incomplete coverage— the main reasons given by people who "tried" but did not buy—make perfect sense. Because it has lower administrative cost and commands a tax subsidy, group insurance is cheaper than individual insurance for the great bulk of the population. And because it is cheaper—artificially so, because of the tax subsidy— people buy more of it.[5] Thus the survey's main finding that people with individual insurance pay more and get less than people with group insurance is no surprise. Criticizing individual coverage in this context is like criticizing Cinderella for poor fashion sense: given the more adverse circumstances in the individual market, the people who cannot find a group alternative do the best they can, but that outcome has to be inferior to group insurance. It is surely possible to find an individual product with low cost-sharing and highly permissive managed care, but it is so expensive that people generally do not choose it.

So the poor relative performance of this market is understandable. The study's conclusion is not. The conclusion is that "the individual market in its current form does not provide a viable alternative to employer-based coverage." That is true enough for people who have an employer-based alternative, but for the great bulk of people in the individual market, there is no such alterna-

---

5. Group insurance premiums can be excluded from workers' taxable incomes and thus receive a tax subsidy that is generally not available to those who buy individual coverage.

tive that they find attractive. (In principle, anyone could take a job at a company providing group coverage, such as Starbucks, but that may not be the preferred employment option for most.) For these people, their only practical option is individual coverage or no coverage. For them, as long as their income is not at the poverty level, at least some type of individual policy (even if only catastrophic coverage with a high deductible but a low premium) is a viable option. I would agree with another conclusion of the study—that the individual market "is inadequate as a source of affordable health insurance coverage for those without access to employer-based coverage," if "inadequate" refers to the "high unsubsidized price" (Commonwealth Fund 2009, 9). But then the solution should be an effort to get the administrative cost down and subsidies equalized so this poor stepsister in the insurance market can at least make a reasonable showing at the ball.

One other conclusion of the study—that those with health problems were "least likely" to "find an individual plan that meets their needs" is misleading, since other data analyses using larger samples of better data show that higher risks are often as likely or more likely to get individual coverage than lower risks (though, of course, they might have preferred much more generous coverage than they chose given the price they faced). Finally, the study clearly shows that overinsurance—a large number of people choosing subsidized coverage with zero deductibles and minimal cost-sharing—is a serious problem with employer-based coverage, and to a much greater extent than with individual coverage. Nearly a third of people had coverage with zero deductibles.[6]

The high proportion of disappointed potential buyers in the Commonwealth study is not a consistent finding. A recent study by America's Health Insurance Plans (AHIP) of nearly two million applicants for individual insurance showed that only 10% were excluded from coverage by medical underwriting and that, of those offered coverage, more people were offered discounts from standard coverage risk rates that were uprated (2007). The 2007 Commonwealth study in contrast asked only about those charged more, not about those charged less. That study did not say what proportion of those who got as far as underwriting then accepted the offered coverage, nor what proportion of the potential customer base got as far as applying to be underwritten. An earlier case study by the National Association of Health Underwriters (NAHU) found that almost every potential buyer even with a chronic condition was eventually able to get an insurance offer if they persisted in searching among companies despite being rejected at first application (2002).

---

6. The Commonwealth study found that 36% of those who "tried to buy" were either rejected for coverage or charged a higher premium.

Lowering administrative costs

Individual insurance is expensive for a reason: its administrative costs per insured person are high. Only a revolutionary shift to a single-payer system or futuristic methods for electronic claims processing could affect this cost, and that is not likely to happen nationwide any time soon. Moreover, the often-quoted 2% to 3% figure for administrative costs for the conventional Medicare coverage is necessarily lower than the cost of claim processing in a private market, because (among other reasons) private insurers do not have Medicare's ability to convert questionable provider reimbursement behavior into a federal offense, and because Medicare's research, development, and lobbying costs are not charged off as insurer administrative expenses. Costs for selling, underwriting, billing, and general administration that vary substantially across insurance types are also important. The loading percentage is also lowered by the substantially larger dollar volume of Medicare claims per beneficiary.

So let us take it as given that the cost of individual insurance will be relatively high but that the uninsured people we want to reach will be making individual voluntary choices whether or not to take insurance *and* that at least initially they will be charged the full price for that insurance. If individual insurance is the only feasible game in town, is there any way to lower the cost of reaching them?

Buying groups and exchanges: How many Chihuahuas equal a Great Dane?

There have been many attempts to obtain lower administrative costs for individuals and small employers by creating larger buying groups or exchanges. It is crucial to note that participation in these groups, as well as the decision to offer insurance, had (before the advent of the Massachusetts Connector) been voluntary. These entities contract with a subset of all possible insurers, communicate information about premiums, and often then help to collect premiums from people who agree to get their coverage in this way.

The key elements of an exchange, according to Kingsdale and Bertko (2009), are that it is organized by government and that it is separate from alternative ways (if permitted) in which people can get individual or small-group insurance. Within these broad limits, there are models of varying degrees of exchange intrusiveness: from functioning just to list premium and policy characteristics for all licensed insurers in a market, through voluntary buying groups in which firms participating in the exchange have advantages in getting the buying group's business, to having the exchange itself bargain with insurers, regulate coverage and payment methods, and set premiums.

Voluntary buying groups have the longest record. I do not believe there is a single example of permanent success with voluntary buying groups here. The reason

51

for failure is ominous and obvious: whatever the size and configuration of the voluntary entity of which the buyer becomes a part, the buyer still must choose individually or as a small firm to belong to and operate through the large group in the exchange. The buyer (individual or small firm) does not shed skepticism, inertia, and apprehension just by joining or participating in this entity; he or she will be subject to the same kind of selling job an individual customer would be subject to. Once snared, the member might be handled at lower cost in an exchange or buying group (though the two-stage process may have duplicative costs of its own), but even here there may still need to be individual care and feeding and, compared to real group insurance, each person must explicitly pay the full premium if there is no subsidy.

There are then few a priori reasons to expect substantial economies of scale in administrative costs from exchanges. So then what might make voluntary "groups of individuals" work better in the future? One approach might involve new technology. There may be ways to lower the cost of searching for coverage, informing one's self about the options, actually applying, and then paying premiums on a continuous basis. The advent of electronic methods for transacting creates some hope here. Research suggests that online insurance purchasing has lowered administrative cost and increased competition for some other kinds of insurance, such as life insurance.

Web-based health insurance offerings have emerged, and have had some success in terms of their volume, though little apparent effect on the total number of un-insured. There is some research on the potential advantages here, based on comparing information on actual premiums paid in the pre-e-insurance period with the premiums quoted on websites. That information is somewhat mixed. Under reasonable assumptions about the cost trend, it seems that the pre-Web premiums people actually paid were lower than the *average* premiums quoted on the Web, especially for older and presumably higher risks (Pauly, Herring, and Song 2006). So just going to a website, selecting an insurer at random, and contemplating buying is not going to yield a premium appreciably below that yielded by the traditional process.

Upon reflection, this may be not much of a surprise. Before the web, people used brokers to search and, though the brokers required commissions, buyers were benefited by being channeled to insurers with lower overall prices, based on the broker's previous higher volume of searches. This alternative intensive search process would have been most rational for higher risks who had more to lose from overpaying for insurance, and indeed the research suggests that the average Web premiums were a worse deal for older risks.

A somewhat more optimistic outcome is possible if we assume that people would choose not the average premium plan on the Web but the lowest (or at least a relatively low) quote. Then there is some evidence of savings, but the savings at best are quite modest. Probably the reason is that the underwriting, and the exchange of information, still needs to be done largely offline on a personal basis; the selling is not yet totally "routinized," like booking an airline ticket or paying credit card bills online, perhaps for reasons we will explore further below. Online insurance is still a boutique product; no all-electronic product has as yet emerged.

If the Web or neighborhood insurance broker cannot be that much of a better deal on individual health insurance, can we expect that some type of quasi-group arrangement will do better? Here there is (as always) hope for the future, but little evidence of past success. Exchanges simply pass through administrative costs (such as broker commissions), but they may allow buyers to more easily determine which sellers have lower administrative costs and lower target profits. Here again, we have hopes, but not evidence. By encouraging or requiring insurers to post premiums in a common and organized setting, some of the troublesome price dispersion already noted might be mitigated. It is less obvious that average administrative costs will be lowered.

Massachusetts set up the Connector as an exchange-type vehicle for making coverage available to people who sought insurance as members of small employment-based groups, or as individuals, as a setting for enforcing rules about how such coverage could be sold, and as an institutional arrangement for subsidizing coverage for those judged unable to afford insurance premiums. Has this arrangement improved the individual insurance market? The main finding here is that premiums in this market are judged to be significantly lower than the former average premium for individual insurance in Massachusetts. Of course, Massachusetts was one of the most expensive states in the country for individual insurance before the creation of the exchange, due to a combination of high medical expenses and adverse selection resulting from community rating in its individual market.

The evidence is not yet complete that would allow us to divide up the causes, but part of the reason for the lower premiums in the exchange is that its benchmark affordable plan involved higher cost-sharing than had previously prevailed; an amusing story in the Boston papers explained how the Blue Cross plan reacted to a demand from the group planning health reform for a lower premium by finding a way to cut the premium—by cutting coverage! Somewhat more speculatively, the combination of new subsidies and new penalties for noncoverage probably caused some low risks to seek coverage, thus lowering the average community-rated premium. It is possible that this lower premium is an example of a kind of low-level equilibrium under adverse selection.

The exchange almost surely provided benefit in some other ways. It did make it easier for people to shop across insurers for a better deal (although the effect of this feature on average premiums paid is hard to separate out). It probably was associated with lower administrative costs, but these cost savings almost surely were caused by the subsidy/mandate combination prompting people to seek coverage, not by economies of administration, per se. In fact, broker commissions continued to be permitted in the exchange. Another potentially useful feature of the Massachusetts plan was a requirement that employers set up Section 125 ("cafeteria") plans even if there was no employer contribution, thus allowing all workers to get a tax exclusion for worker premium contributions, but apparently no one has used this path.

The best part of the idea of an exchange is to reduce buyer search costs by standardizing the most popular policy options and bringing together a number of insurers to propose premiums on the exchange. However, this approach has so far only been used in states that do not allow explicit underwriting of coverage; it would be more challenging to offer better information on prices for standardized coverage when insurers are also adjusting the risk levels they accept to the premiums they charge. And we do not really know whether on balance buyers ended up with better deals—only that, whatever they paid, at least it came from an apparently tidy market.

The other potential benefit from an exchange is a benefit of individual insurance now: insurance obtained in the exchange would be portable across jobs. The main novelty here is that very-small-group insurance essentially is transformed into individual insurance. Since I have argued that individual insurance does have some positive features, I regard this change as one for the better. One question is whether the tax and possibly some of the other advantages of group insurance can still be reaped in a setting where the insurance itself is owned and paid for by the individual, not the group or the employer. We still do not know the answer to this question.

Exchanges now being seriously discussed (or recently created) have not been mild attempts to improve market function; instead, some versions, including that used by Massachusetts, have come with a heavy overburden of premium and product regulation. It is this propensity for dysfunctional regulation that sours the concept of an exchange. The primary regulatory goal is community rating, and the consequences of attempts to enforce community-rating rules can be adverse.

As already noted, the main downside is that, because of a rule requiring insurers to charge the same premium for the same policy to all, incentives for adverse selection and cream-skimming are created where they did not need to exist. Any opportunity for choice across insurance policies then raises the opportunity for adverse selection, which undoes risk transfers and may destroy the entire market. To attempt to prevent this, regulators are inexorably led to rule out offering lower-coverage policies because those policies might pick off the low risks. Never mind that they might also be good for average risks who are only moderately risk averse but very concerned about moral hazard, and never mind that innovation overall may be stifled. At least low risks are not avoiding their obligation to make transfers to high risks. As one member of the Massachusetts board said, "allowing people to pick and choose . . . undermines broad spreading of risk" (Turnbull 2009). At present, high-deductible plans are included in the exchange, but the future for this concession to Republicans cannot be regarded as very bright.

Finally, regulators are human. They develop affection for some policy designs and abhor others. Try as they might, they fall prey to a soft paternalism in which they want to channel people toward particular policy designs. These sentiments creep into the rules. The argument that people have too many choices, that options should be standardized yet further to allow more efficient shopping, feeds into these urges.

Does this kind of heavy-handed regulation actually occur? According to Charlie Baker, it has occurred in Massachusetts. The state had to define "minimum creditable coverage," and in so doing it both retained every mandated benefit that had previously been lobbied into existence and added a requirement for outpatient drug coverage. It also imposed maxima on deductibles ($2,000 for individuals, no matter what assets they held or what attitude they had toward risk) and out-of-pocket payments ($5,000 for an individual). The state is also proposing to mandate new bundled ways to pay for health care that are both revolutionary and untried, although that policy is probably not the consequence of the exchange mechanism but rather is borne of quiet desperation as medical spending, already much above average in Massachusetts, has continued to grow even as the uninsured are covered and supposedly are now getting the needed preventive care that saves on health care costs.

The problem here is not that these rules themselves raised costs directly, since (especially with the tax subsidy and other subsidies) most people want more generous coverage than the minimum. But in economic theory even a relatively small minority of people with strong incentives to be aggressive shoppers keeps down the cost for all, and yet regulation may prevent them from playing this role.

On balance, does the Massachusetts exchange represent a model for a national plan (even one that imagines federally required but state-run exchanges)? As already noted, many questions still cannot be answered. We know that the overall Massachusetts plan reduced the fraction of uninsured in that state, and we know that the subsidies that were effective in doing this are increasingly straining the state's budget, but we do not know what would have happened without subsidies, specification of minimum qualified plans, penalties for no insurance, or requirements for a Section 125 offering, without an exchange. There is no evidence of an equally dramatic drop in individual insurance administrative cost in Massachusetts beyond what subsidization itself would have generated. To score savings for the exchange per se the administrative cost percentage would have to be pushed below 15% for individual insurance, and that has not yet happened. It is also important to remember that much of the regulation and organization embodied in the exchange was already present in Massachusetts, one of the distinct minority of states that has found rate regulation (and many other kinds of health care regulation) economically and politically feasible. In a state with lower incomes, more minorities, and less of a tradition of competent regulation, the exchange concept will be more severely challenged.

Regulation and pricing without exchanges

In the absence of a formal exchange or an exchange-like arrangement by a dominant employer, how do people buy small-group or individual insurance? In the status quo, there is some regulation. As already noted, individual coverage is required by current law to be guaranteed renewable at class average rates, there are some guaranteed issue provisions, and in a small number of states the variation in the premium charged to a new (not renewing) insured is regulated with respect to limits on variation with risk. In the small-group market there are no guaranteed renewability provisions applying to individual workers or to individual workers in groups, but premium variation across groups is limited to some extent in the great majority of states, usually with rating "bands" (that is, premiums for any one group cannot be more than twice the average). HIPAA rules do generally require that people insured at one firm who switch jobs be covered at the new firm (if it offers coverage) regardless of risk, but this does not apply to some small firms and, as noted, offers no protection in the individual market. When risk variation is limited, usually variation related to demographics and location is allowed, but not variation based on the prevalence of chronic conditions or health status of a workforce. However, even in heavily regulated states, premiums can vary over time based on past group experience (for example, New York allows experience-rated groups); the rules apply to the initial offering and also depend to some extent on the size of the group, with larger groups having more "credibility" applied to their claims experience. In some states, very small groups are lumped together with individual insurance.

Buyers approach unregulated markets in several potentially different ways. One option is to search online; there are websites for individual insurance and small-group plans, indicating both premiums and coverage. However, anyone seeking to buy what is on the website must apply for coverage and be approved and underwritten—so a listing on a site is not really an unconditional offer to sell at that price. Some individuals and many small employers use brokers, middlemen who gather information about the prices and features of different plans, offer advice to the buyers, and help guide the application and underwriting process. If a broker arranges a transaction, the insurer pays an initial commission (and often a small commission at renewal). The payment system is similar to the way travel agents used to function, who were paid by the airlines rather than, as at present, getting an add-on to the seller's price. Finally, buyers can approach the market in a less organized way, contacting specific companies based on word-of-mouth information or name recognition, with at best an informal search.

The evidence on efficiency of price search under existing arrangements, as noted above, is mixed. There is wide variation in premiums posted or quoted by different insurance companies for apparently similar policies (Pollitz and Sorian 2001), but that is less relevant than information about the variation in prices people actually pay (Pauly, Herring, and Song 2006). Neither the use of the internet nor the use of brokers appears to be sufficient to squeeze out all transactions' price variation (Sood et al. 2004).

The other unique dimension of transaction price variation in this market is whether, at a given price, a seller is willing to underwrite a buyer. It is very clear that different insurers target different risk segments of the markets. Some target to sell only to the best or "cleanest" risks, charging low premiums but rejecting many applicants for what seem minor blemishes in their health records (much to the irritation of the applicants and policymakers). But the rational strategy for the rejected applicant is to continue to search until he or she matches with an insurer whose premium/underwriting target fits that person's risk profile. The evidence is strong that even a relatively tarnished or high risk can get coverage if he or she persists in searching (NAHU 2002). And some of the observed variation in transactions premiums probably reflects this subtle variation across insurers in what they think predicts risk.

So in the end the individual market may not work all that poorly—but it is both bothersome and maddening to buyers. Brokers help, but their inherent conflict of interest (they get paid by the insurer, not the buyer) means that prices do not converge. Of course, if more efficient searching were that valuable, one might imagine that other agents—financial advisors—would emerge to help, and some have. Still, this looks like a terrible way to run a railroad—or a market.

What is the fundamental problem here? Since technological and organizational fixes for high administrative costs are problematic, is there any other way to lower the cost of persuading people to buy insurance? Here we need to go deeper and try to understand why such costly persuasion is necessary. In terms of abstract economic theory, insurance is desirable because it allows risk-averse people to be better off, to have higher "expected utility," as they reduce the risk of a very high and financially crippling medical bill. But if insurance is as good a thing as we think, why should people have to be talked into it? For many other products, selling costs are modest. I volunteer to go to the supermarket to get food for tonight's dinner, even bearing some costs to get there; I do not have to be persuaded. To be sure, there are some products that famously have to be "sold": soft drinks or ready-to-eat cereals are products with high selling costs as a proportion of sales. But neither of these are products that fulfill a fundamental human need or desire. If we know why (or whether) health insurance has to be sold rather than bought, perhaps that can point the way toward methods to reduce costs. The answer to this question depends, in large part, on the premium charged for coverage relative to the benefits the insured expects to collect, but it also depends on buyer information and insurer transparency. We look at the price-availability issue first, and then move on to consider other factors.

Insurance company economics, sharp practices, premiums, and exclusions

Insurers vary in the premiums they charge and the policies they follow in deciding to issue insurance to new policyholders. One often-criticized feature of insurance, especially individual insurance, is a preexisting-condition exclusion. This feature applies only to uninsured people seeking insurance or those who are newly insured. As a condition of coverage, insurers may exclude benefit payment for some period of time for conditions the person could reasonably have known about before coverage or for care in a current episode of treatment. Thus, if I knew I had an allergy (usually because a doctor told me so and/or because I sought care for it), treatment might not be covered for a period generally ranging from nine months to two years. Or if I was in the middle of treatment for some symptoms (even if I did not yet have a diagnosis), future care in that course of treatment would not be covered. The rationale for exclusion is that the purpose of insurance is to pay for uncertain events, not those that are already known to exist. In the extreme case, were there no such exclusions allowed, people would not buy insurance until they got sick, but then the premiums needed to cover their costs would be very high because they could not be averaged over people who did not get sick. Obviously, a policy with no exclusions at all would be very expensive, but there is choice among firms with a variety of different exclusion policies. Different companies currently apply these exclusions with different degrees of strictness (and for different periods of time). Less strict exclusion rules are matched by higher premiums.

Why do people seek or accept policies that have these exclusions? The answer that insurers require them is not satisfactory, since insurers will offer anything consumers are willing to pay for; consumer acceptance is also required. An alternative strategy for insurers would be to agree to cover everything, but to (upwardly) risk-adjust premiums to deal with the presence of chronic conditions—and such adjustment does occur to a fairly significant extent for new insurance applicants. The exclusions are present as a secondary device to deal with risk variation and attendant possible adverse selection; they reflect the practical idea that premiums cannot be adjusted for everything and insurers might not find it worthwhile to discover everything about risk in advance. Despite their recent publicity, these exclusions affect very few people and often have modest effects when they do.

But they bother people a lot. There is a chance that an exclusion exposes a person to a large bill. Perhaps part of the reason is that a person who initially chose a plan with stricter rules to save just a few dollars on premiums is frustrated if those rules end up affecting that person when the prior condition does flare up again. It is the frustration of a gamble gone wrong. What also bothers people is having to argue with the insurance company, should they get sick soon after getting new coverage. The point to be made here is that you can reduce frustration and argument by paying more. Consumers may well have a hard time knowing which companies follow which policies (especially if they do not use a knowledgeable independent agent or financial advisor), and so there may be some case for defining a standard set of provisions. And, as those experts know, some companies, even some large insurers, have a reputation for being more likely to engage in sharp practices. Everyone who applies or who files a claim after having just begun insurance coverage will be asked about the possible preexisting nature of the illness, and everyone who is asked will be irritated by the question. Finally, even companies with middle-of-the-road policies will from time to time be overly aggressive in individual cases. In effect, the exclusion causes people to suffer administrative costs and even lack coverage on a basis that is doubly unpredictable—depending on whether the person gets sick and what their company then does.

The problem is clear. We would rather avoid this bothersome lottery, but doing so completely would make insurance less attractive to most people most of the time (since most people at any point in time are not sick or suffering a chronic condition) and unaffordable when they did seek it. Trying to deal with what is presently a very minor problem even in the individual market (though occasionally serious for the rare household) runs the real risk of creating a much more serious problem of bad incentives for healthy people thinking of (not) buying insurance. A minor flaw could be turned into a catastrophe. And, as we shall see, there are better ways than prohibition to deal with the few high risks who would be caught by exclusions.

So why are such forms of "insurance reform" apparently popular with policymakers? Anger at insurance companies appeals to the inner lawyer (or locker-room liberal) in all of us, but not all exclusions should be prohibited. There is a temptation to insurance fraud; public-interest radio spots in Philadelphia have been warning people about buying auto insurance and then making claims for "pre-existing collisions." Insurance is complex, and, having paid a premium, we all want to collect as much as we can and are upset when insurers turn down even those claims we thought that policy provisions made them unlikely to pay. Some compromise, and an adult attitude, is needed as long as some people are sometimes uninsured because insurance purchase is voluntary.

Here is how to think about the trade-off. If there were no exclusions and no waiting periods, virtually all people who became high risks would probably end up with coverage (as long as they could raise the money for the very high insurance premiums), but virtually all low risks would decline that very expensive insurance. As we allow exclusions or make the time we have to wait to get insurance longer, some high-risk people and high-risk conditions will be dropped out but more low-risk people and their illnesses will be covered. What is the right balance?

The answer to that question depends in part on social values: how much does it bother me for a low-risk person to be without coverage, and how much for a high-risk person? Since we drive away more low risks for every high risk we bring in, even if we feel worse about uninsured high risks than low risks, we still have a judgment call to make. Another kind of judgment call concerns exclusions versus waiting periods for coverage to begin. The trade-off is that an exclusion exposes the person to risk for the designated condition but provides immediate coverage for all other services, while a waiting period denies coverage for everything for some period of time. Usually the exclusion period is longer than the waiting period—but the waiting period is worse regarding access to care.

Some combination of incentives to get insurance before you get sick—exclusions not based on "gotcha" clauses but properly targeted at things people should have anticipated, plus relatively brief waiting periods—might provide the best balanced incentive for coverage and care. Insurers sometimes and insurance critics frequently fall prey to the notion that denying legitimate claims, or slipping out of them in some way, is the path to high long-run profits. But in reality insurers have no principles about what claims they will or will not pay; as long as the buyer is willing to pay a high enough premium and the policy language can be clear, insurers would be willing to pay for whatever buyers want— experimental treatment, ongoing illnesses, aromatherapy, and others. (Consider the Nationwide auto insurance policy that promises not to raise your premium if you have an accident; sounds great, but that insurance is therefore more expensive upfront than strictly experience-rated coverage.) The evidence is that consumers are not really willing to pay for soft-hearted but expensive health insurance policies but then get frustrated when the rules kick in. We definitely do not yet know enough to mandate any particular policy, so at least some flexibility—with prohibitions on the arbitrary and unreasonable, probably limiting aggressive insurer behavior more for lower-income people—might be the best way to go. Heavy-handed blanket prohibitions motivated more by political sound-bite appeal than by good sense would not be good.

The answer also depends on what else we do about high risks. If there is an alternative for high risks to conventional coverage with exclusions (for example, somewhat more expensive coverage in a high-risk pool), then there is less need to prohibit exclusions in conventional coverage. It is interesting that in unregulated markets, waiting periods are rare and brief (if coverage is delayed, it is usually for only a month or so), but exclusions are common, though usually limited to two years or less. The market test would suggest that waiting periods are inferior to exclusions, but the former probably benefit higher risks somewhat more than the latter. But in unregulated markets, high risks can often get complete coverage for all conditions right away if they are willing to pay a high-risk premium, something precluded under community rating. On the other hand, an uninsured person with a high-risk condition could be sure of getting coverage under a waiting period (just by waiting long enough), whereas the condition might be permanently excluded under the exclusion model. But this almost never happens, except for rare high-cost conditions (for example, hemophilia or cystic fibrosis) because exclusions have time limits as well. Still another compromise is to give buyers an option to take coverage at a given point in time but then charge them a higher premium in the future if they decline their first chance.

Whether the deterrent to being an uninsured high risk is the possibility of an exclusion or a waiting period, the best arrangement would be for consumers to take coverage beforehand with guaranteed renewability. The more regulation requires insurers to be permissive in accepting people with prior conditions, the less likely this is to happen. There needs to be a trade-off here as well. Some combination of penalty for being uninsured and additional penalty for being high-risk uninsured should be part of the mix. The more effective these incentives, the less effort needs to be put into monitoring cream-skimming and limiting policy designs that appeal to low risks—precisely because coverage should appeal to low risks. It may well be that excluding conditions is not the best way to offer an incentive to take coverage when healthy. What is important here, then, is not the principle but the practice.

Subsidies

The simplest version of the insurance-decision process explains why a subsidy, even a modest one, can be highly effective in stimulating coverage (an obvious result) *and* in lowering administrative costs (a less obvious result) *and* in reducing risk rating, exclusions, or waiting periods (an even less obvious result). The fundamental idea is simple: in deciding on insurance, the person compares the insurance premium to the out-of-pocket expenses expected to be incurred in the absence of insurance, estimating the latter (in the economics version of the story) by weighting each possible expenditure by the subjective probability that it will happen. If this expected value of the benefits from the insurance policy is less than (or even close to) the premium paid for the policy, the person will undoubtedly gain from buying the policy and will buy it. If the premium remains low relative to the expected value of benefits, the person will be eager to pay the bill for the renewal premium as well.

The reason why many do not buy individual health insurance is that they believe (whether correctly or not) that the premium is high relative to their expected benefit. It is not that they do not think insurance is valuable, or even that they could not, if pressed, come up with the premium; it is that they do not think it is a good deal for what they have to pay for it.

Why might so many think this? For one thing, because it is often true. The loading that typically prevails in individual insurance is high, and there is no tax subsidy. So on average, people who buy individual health insurance to cover a given prospective set of possible medical expenses will spend a lot more than the average expense of those who take a chance without insurance. Put slightly differently, compared to shelling out high premiums for individual insurance, most people who remain uninsured will be better off financially at the end of the year; the benefits they get back would be less than the premium they paid. Most people will not get very sick and will not make money off their insurance, and so they may regard it as a poor investment.

However, people who are risk-averse enough will be willing to pay a premium that is high relative to benefits rather than risk the chance of an expense much higher than the premium. One does not buy insurance because it is a good investment; one buys it because it helps enormously in the unlikely event of being unlucky in health. (The level of loading that prevails in the individual health insurance market is similar to that in the individual life insurance market, and the takeup rate in both markets is similar, so we probably do not want to go too far in suggesting more novel theories for nonpurchase. The loading is also similar to that in homeowners and automobile collision insurance, but in these cases there are insurance requirements from lenders that, for people with a mortgage or who are paying off their car over time, assure a high-proportion purchasing.)

Still, there is some evidence that people underestimate their expected losses for health care; this is especially true of younger people who think they will almost never need medical care. There is also some evidence that people believe individual health insurance to be more expensive than it really is and so never even bother to search.

Some aggressive strategies for convincing people that they are at risk, that health insurance is a reasonably good value, and that they should be worried about risk, appear to be only moderately successful. Although some insurers have pushed such plans ("Tonik" in California), most have not, and low risks remain uncovered. An alternative and more effective strategy to induce coverage is to lower the explicit price paid for insurance; that is, to offer a "subsidized" price and so make the loading be negative. Then the takeup of insurance is so attractive that few resources need to be expended to convince people in the first place or to get them to renew. The subsidy could be paid by others (taxpayers, other insureds), or it might even be paid by recipients in the form of a compulsory contribution to insurance premiums. The key point is that if the explicit premium the buyer could avoid paying by declining coverage can be made less than the full premium, buyers will not need costly persuasion. The best way to persuade people to buy insurance is to make it less expensive; even "young immortals" will buy at a low enough price.

Lower price is part of the secret of success in group (especially large group) insurance. The worker eligible for such coverage now is usually charged an explicit premium that he could avoid by declining to take the group insurance. But this premium is only a small fraction

(20%–25%) of the total premium and therefore looks reasonable (even relative to the low individual premium for young workers); almost all workers therefore take offered coverage.

But workers pay for the other part of the premium by accepting lower money wages (Pauly 1997). Why do they agree to this kind of trick or precommitment, rather than waiting to decide on paying, or not paying, the full premium for coverage? Tax subsidies are one major part of the reason. But another part may be that workers trust the insurance through their job to be a reasonably good buy most of the time. They anticipate that they might sometimes make mistakes in evaluating insurance if they were to do so themselves. Precommiting a major share of the premium so that it will be rational to drop coverage only in the rare case when its value drops below 25% of its premium may be a good compromise, one that avoids the need to revisit the insurance-purchase decision every year.

What to hope for and what to expect

There is already voluntary private insurance with the premium subsidized at the point of purchase that might tell us what would happen were individual insurance markets subsidized. Specifically, large-group insurance achieves two of the three objectives posed above. In particular, it has low loading costs, estimated to be as low as 5% of premiums for very large groups. This means that little is wasted on pure insurance administration, and it compares favorably with administrative cost percentages in Medicare and Medicaid. It is also attractive enough because of the tax subsidy to have a very high participation rate among eligibles, almost always above 90%.

Here is another example of subsidized insurance and its loading cost: Chile compels workers to devote a portion of their payroll tax to health insurance but permits them to elect a private individual insurance option. These "ISAPRE" insurances have loadings of about half those of individual health insurance in the United States, at about 14% (in 2007). The reason is not that the Chileans are much more efficient at the insurance business than the Americans are; the reason, rather, is that in Chile the insurance companies only have to guide the choice of which kind of insurance to take, not make the hard sell that some kind of insurance is better than being totally uninsured.

In an historical example in the United States, regulation for a time forced the near-monopolistic Blue Cross plan of New Jersey to cross-subsidize the individual market; with this subsidy, the administrative cost of individual health insurance was also only about 14% of premiums.

The point here is that a subsidy does more than increase the takeup at a given loading; it actually permits a dramatic reduction in loading itself because it reduces the cost of persuading people to take coverage. Subsidized insurance is more efficient with regard to administrative cost because of a kind of self-fulfilling prophecy: by making premiums more attractive, selling costs can be lowered, but at lower selling costs, attractive premiums can eventually become financially feasible.

This powerful point, which I believe is not well recognized either in the health policy or the insurance economics literature, has two important implications, one fairly obvious and the other less so. The obvious implication is that with a subsidy, the specific administrative arrangement for insurance becomes both less important and less of a factor in takeup. For example, the Massachusetts Connector may well have relatively low administrative cost, but so would almost any other way of administering insurance given that state's large subsidy to people with incomes below 300% of poverty and its penalty for uninsurance to others. It is not the whole bundle of features of a high-performance (and high-regulation) health system that lowers individual insurance administrative cost; the active ingredient is the subsidy. A system with only brokers or agents would also be cheap, because they would not have as much work to do in persuading people to take coverage as they did in the pre-subsidy market. The use of an online website might also work quite well.

The best policy (though not the one followed in Massachusetts) might be to offer subsidies especially targeted at buyers with lower insurance demand, but then let consumers choose in a neutral way how they want to obtain insurance. They might well want to use an insurance exchange, but they might actually prefer other methods—for example, the direct use of brokers or agents who know them personally and can offer better advice to the inexperienced buyer than the neutral and impersonal exchange. The Connector is analogized to a stock exchange, but many people who use the stock exchange use a broker or investment advisor, and the stock exchange itself provides no investment advice. The distinctions in reality between an insurance exchange and the more typical individual market with brokers and agents are easy to overstate; it is most likely that most consumers will not obtain their insurance without assistance, just as many small investors do not use low-service discount stockbrokers.

The less obvious point is that lowering price with a subsidy might even lower administrative costs so much as to eliminate (or at least greatly reduce) the need for a subsidy. More formally, there may be a break-even equilibrium at a low insurance premium with high volume, but markets may currently be trapped in another equilibrium with high premiums and low volume. Table 4 shows an example.

The first row roughly reproduces the current situation in the individual insurance market. The second row shows a hypothetical increase in quantity demanded when explicit premiums are cut by a third.

If sellers of insurance are rational profit maximizers,

TABLE 4
How a Subsidy Might Lower Administrative Loading
as a Percentage of Premiums

Total Loading	Selling Cost	Other Cost	Subsidy	% Buying
30%	22%	8%	0	25%
10%	7%	8%	(–5%)	80%

they have presumably chosen their current (high) level of selling effort because, were they to reduce selling costs, commissions, and the like, the money they would save by so doing is more than offset by the reduction in net revenues they would expect from selling insurance, as buyers would disappear; the current position of high costs, low quantity, but high prices paid by those few buyers remaining in the market is a "local profit-maximizing equilibrium." Suppose selling costs were greatly reduced, but price was also lowered considerably. That lower price might bring forth enough demand to cover the remaining costs and to counteract the consequences of reduced persuasion, thereby leading to enough revenue. We could imagine price being close to the actuarially fair premium plus the small (and constant-over-units) claims-processing costs. There might be many people who would seek out insurance at that low price, thus permitting insurers to cover their cost without even a subsidy, or without much of a subsidy.

The key parameters here are the response of quantity

demanded, given selling costs, to premium, and the response of quantity demanded, given premium, to selling costs—in elasticity terms, the price and selling-cost elasticities of demand. The well-known Dorfman-Steiner theorem states that if these two elasticities are given and constant, the amount of selling expense will be greater the higher the selling cost elasticity relative to the price elasticity (in absolute value). But it is possible that the selling cost elasticity is lower at low levels of selling cost than at high levels; if so, there may be more than one local equilibrium.

More concretely, jumping to a "mass marketed" insurance plan, priced low and sold with low-cost selling methods, might be profitable (or require only a modest subsidy)—even if a slightly lower-priced and a slightly less intensively marketed plan than the current one is not. This hope is buoyed by noting an important precedent: auto insurance. Both third-party and collision insurance used to be sold primarily by the American agency system, using brokers and agents paid high commissions and leading to high premiums and high loadings. Then, first Allstate and, subsequently and more aggressively, GEICO pioneered the "direct writer" system, in which agents were salaried or nonexistent; general advertising was substituted for individual house calls; and toll-free phone numbers were used to communicate with potential customers, quote premiums, and complete applications. No government had to create an exchange. The same phenomenon might apply to individual health insurance, especially since a low premium might draw into the market people less interested in intensive service from their insurance and more interested in low price and value. Costco on the West Coast has been experimenting with an in-store sales system similar to what Allstate used in its early, Sears-owned stage. It offers individual health insurance to "Costco Executive Members" through the Pacificare plan, payable by electronic funds transfer from the insured's bank account.

Economic theorists are concerned that adverse selection might limit the size of the individual market, and policymakers are concerned about risk rating. In reality, individual insurance markets in states without premium regulation do not appear to be in an adverse selection equilibrium, selling insurance at high premiums to a few high risks. Instead, the usual criticism is just the reverse: individual insurers without regulation sell only to very healthy low risks at what must be a relatively low premium and moderately high loading, with some part of loading representing the cost of underwriting to screen out higher risks. (The argument that community rating will reduce the net numbers of uninsured by making insurance more affordable to high risks is, as already discussed above, just wrong.) The explicit cost of underwriting in individual insurance already appears to be a small fraction of premiums; probably some of the agents' commission is for informal screening and channeling as well. But if insurance were subsidized modestly, so that more lower risks were attracted into insurance markets, it would not pay for insurers to underwrite as vigorously as they do now. The purpose of costly underwriting is to identify the high-risk applicants, but underwriting requires that every applicant be reviewed. It only makes sense to spend resources on a careful review if you think there is a large enough fraction of applicants you would want to decline. If subsidies enrich the pool of applicants with many more good risks, it becomes much less cost effective to screen, and so screening efforts will decline. It would also no longer pay as much for low risks to search aggressively for policies with premiums tied to their risk levels, if high risks are not segmented out.

Regardless of the current situation, a modest subsidy might change things. It might permit firms to cover the costs of the small number of high risks and still be attractive to the much larger number of moderate-to-low risks. And if insurers know that, at this modestly subsidized premium, their pool of applicants will contain a very small proportion of high risks and a very large proportion of eager moderate-to-low risks, it will not even be worthwhile to spend substantial resources to screen many applicants just to identify a few high risks.

Guaranteed renewability also limits adverse selection now, and could be improved to virtually eliminate it over time. The reason why guaranteed renewability is adverse-selection-proof is that good risks are always charged a premium they find attractive in a guaranteed-renewability contract. Hence, there is no way an outside insurer can pick them off. Those who have become high risks are obviously delighted to be in their guaranteed-renewability contract and so have little to gain from slipping into other lower-risk pools. Of course, guaranteed renewability is no solution for people who are already high risk and uninsured. There would be a backlog of uninsured high risks to be cleared even if guaranteed renewability is made universal. Guaranteed renewability requires signing people up while they are still healthy and so cannot work with people who have already become high risks at a young age. But the current stock of uninsured truly high risks is actually quite small among young adults; the fraction of young people with birth defects, chronic conditions, or permanent disabilities (as to physical health) is only about three percent of their age group. So, targeted programs (rather than market-wide regulation) are better for dealing with this small minority.

For these initial high risks, some subsidized arrangement would be desirable. It should, as an interim step, take the form of a high-risk pool financed by general revenue taxation; it should not (for reasons discussed earlier) take the form of community rating, rating bands, or prohibition of exclusions.

Let me share a brief comment on the role of high-risk pools in the past and in a reformed system. Such pools have been properly criticized as a weak solution to the problem of uninsured high risks, but they could be made to work better and to function as a fallback in a system

83

that relies on universal guaranteed renewability. Current high-risk pools are not attractive because they cover only a small fraction of high risks, are often financed by taxes or assessments that increase insurance premiums, and sometimes close to new enrollment. But with robust guaranteed renewability, there would be many fewer high risks needing help from a pool; in effect, their current small scale may fit the new environment. High-risk pools are also criticized because they do not more generously subsidize low-income high risks, although most of those low-income households could not afford coverage even at low-risk premiums. The problem here is not the high-risk pool concept per se, or even their management (which appears to be competent), but rather their inadequate budgets. In ideal reform, budgets would be adequate but, as noted, may not need to be so large if guaranteed renewability reduces the need for this arrangement since there would then be few uninsured high risks remaining.

Offering the right product

The third kind of potentially desirable change in the individual health insurance market is related to product design. Given some level of administrative cost and some level of subsidy, the way to maximize the chance that a person will choose to obtain insurance is to offer the person the insurance design that he or she likes best for the money. This sturdy truism is often ignored; policymakers and policy analysts alike endlessly debate what is the best kind of insurance product in their personal opinion, with passionate and conflicting views on high-deductible health plans, managed care, limited out-of-pocket payment, and coverage of preventive care. Much of the reason for the argument is that policymakers have skipped a step: they are trying to specify what coverage consumers should have to get them closer to the care they need. The missing step, of course, is that ideal coverage is only useful if the person has the insurance to begin with, and is able and willing to buy it. The insurance plan that greatly improves one's health, or maximizes one's health for the money, will not affect one's actual health unless one is willing to choose that insurance.

This plain fact suggests a less-than-obvious policy: given some actuarial value, the best way to maximize the chance that a person will buy coverage, given a subsidy (if any), is the policy design that the person likes best, and the best way to make this happen is to let people choose their own options with very light minimum-benefit requirements. The least constraining version of this plan would be to specify an average actuarial value and a subsidy, and allow people to choose whatever insurance they wish, within broad limits, that has an average cost equal to or greater than that value. The lowest-coverage policy might be limited and less than ideal in policymakers' judgment, but at least it would be free and therefore universal.

Even this simple process still leaves open the question of specifying the minimum actuarial value and the subsidy. A program that permitted eligible policies to have premium values very close to the subsidy (so that it would be virtually free) should technically reduce the number of people with literally zero coverage to zero, for who would reject free insurance? But, some might object, such a program would do so only by paying for minimal (or "nonmeaningful") coverage. There needs to be some social decision on the contours of basic coverage, which will probably be different for people at different income levels and possibly vary with other characteristics, such as risk, location, ethnicity, and gender. Efforts to identify coverage considered to satisfy the basic minimum from a societal perspective have not been very successful but must be undertaken. The goal of getting at least some coverage, even if it is not perfect, to everyone is probably preferable to a goal of getting good coverage to only some while leaving others totally unprotected.

There are two other useful policy roles, both generated by the observation that consumers may not all be informed well enough to accurately determine what coverage is indeed best for them. Prohibition of fraudulent or illusory coverage or, more generally, of policy types that no informed person would rationally choose, is a logical extension of standard consumer-product-quality regulation. Less limiting but more sensible may be making the choice of a reasonably good plan the default option or line of least resistance, to nudge people in a decent (even if not the absolute best) direction (Sunstein and Thaler 2008). Even here there can be ambiguities and trade-offs. Suppose an uninsured person is terrified of cancer and therefore foolishly attaches highest value to a policy that paid only for cancer care. It would seem desirable to forbid or discourage this type of coverage on the grounds that it is not rational, yet doing so would involve overriding the citizen's preferences and potentially having the person decide not to take insurance at all. So the hand of regulation should be light and graceful (if that is not too much to ask).

The other potential action is developing new and more attractive insurance designs and making sure they are available in the market. It would seem to be in the business interest of insurance plans themselves to do so, and yet the strongest controversy in the policy sphere has been generated by opinions of third parties about which private plan is "best." Policymakers, physicians, and politicians without expertise in insurance try to decide what insurance people should have—whether HMO, HSA, or prevention-friendly—rather than letting consumers choose for themselves.

One awkward issue here is the dearth of reliable information on whether insurance necessarily causes significantly improved health across the board. There are many correlational studies—people who did not obtain insurance have worse health than those who did—but that correlation may only reflect risky behaviors, including not buying insurance and but also not taking good care of one's self, that distinguish those who did not get insurance from other similar people who did. Studies of the withdrawal of Medicaid show that insurance improves the health of poor children and mothers. We have good evidence on the impact of different policies on medical care use and spending, showing that coverage increases both—since sellers of insurance need to know this in order to price their product. What is lacking is evidence (as opposed to opinion) on what policies have large impacts on health for those not covered by Medicaid—the nonpoor and low-income males. There is a trade-off. Any given level of out-of-pocket spending potentially can (and should, if things are efficient) lead to somewhat lower health status than a policy with higher cost and lower out-of-pocket spending; the slightly lower expected health status is chosen because it is offset by the large savings on total costs. But we do not have any good idea of exactly what degree of health status is traded for how much savings. We cannot with confidence recommend a policy design, for a given premium and/or actuarial value of the total spending, which will lead to a given level of expected health, nor can we say what the target actuarial value should be. Controversy over adequacy and affordability is never-ending and inconclusive because the facts are lacking.

The controversy over the very best study we have— the Rand Health Insurance Experiment—illustrates this problem (Newhouse et al. 1993). In the experiment, higher patient cost-sharing lowered both total spending and the use of medical care that health professionals judged to be essential for health. But, to general surprise, there was no significant relationship between cost-sharing and realized health (except for vision correction) for the great bulk of the study population, with health effects limited to the 6% or so of the population at low income and high initial risk of high blood pressure. How could people who used less care judged to be essential for health end up with no lower levels of health? Perhaps professional judgments are not valid, or perhaps there were offsetting consumer behaviors, but the point is that the current evidence on the linkage between coverage and health outcomes is tangential and imprecise. There are always "concerns" about effects of cost-sharing on health, as in the recent evaluation of consumer-directed health plans (Marquis et al. 2006), but no evidence to judge the health-spending trade-off, and certainly no basis for prohibiting a policy design that some citizens find attractive. I am concerned about many decisions made by my fellow citizens, but that does not mean that I should be able to affect what they do with their own resources (barring evidence for self-harm or serious financial distress).

Data on the effectiveness of different types of care is still quite limited and quite insufficient for coverage design. One needs information on both the value of care and the responsiveness of consumers to coverage. Medical evidence alone is not sufficient.

This absence of good information on the connection between coverage and health suggests in the short run that restrictions on coverage should be light and design should be primarily targeted at attracting people to voluntarily purchase any reasonable health insurance policy and less concerned with their choosing the (as-yet-unknown) precisely "right" level of coverage. Provision of information on the health outcomes associated with different plans may eventually fill the knowledge gap and guide consumers to choose voluntarily the best coverage. We can more usefully worry about "underinsurance" when we get everyone to have some coverage. But in our current state of fairly complete ignorance, we do not want to specify design limits prematurely.

The ideal and the feasible: compromises and mixes

One ideal version of health reform would rely almost entirely on subsidies for low-income average risks, penalties for high-income average risks, and guaranteed renewability to ensure that the population is insured with the right level of insurance. The vision here is one in which the 96% of the population which is good to average risk when they reach the age at which they cease being dependents would all be induced to take coverage with guaranteed renewability at that point. With feasible adjustments to guaranteed renewability to permit people to move across policies when they have good reasons for doing so, all would start with insurance coverage and would be perfectly protected against higher future costs should they become high risk through guaranteed renewability—without side effects and without further compulsion. The tiny fraction of people with disabilities or conditions at young ages could be picked up by existing Medicaid or Medicare programs.

This approach is superior to the high-performance health system relentlessly advocated by some. However, while I believe that serious consideration should be given to implementing this vision and have so argued for many years, some compromises may be necessary, at least for a while until almost everyone has coverage with guaranteed renewability provisions. The most obvious problem is that some people may not, despite our best efforts and best subsidies and penalties, initially take the needed coverage. Then they may become higher risk and need help. Practicality suggests that there must be something in place for this group, some way of limiting the high-risk premium for those people who, through bad luck or bad decisions, somehow end up as sick and uninsured. There is a trade-off here: the more we cushion the consequences of skipping the chance to buy ideal (guaranteed renewable) coverage, the more we distort incentives—both incentives to protect against becoming a high risk and even incentives to becoming insured at all regardless of risk level.

After all, the motivation for consumers to be willing

to pay in advance for a market mechanism to protect against risk reclassification—guaranteed renewability—is the possibility of reclassification. If, at the extreme, health insurance were to be fully community rated and issue is guaranteed without exclusion of coverage for services related to current health status, there is no risk and therefore no motive to get insurance. If rating instead puts bounds on the premiums that can be charged to high risks but allows somewhat higher premiums for them, there will then be a motive for guaranteed renewability, but that motive will be attenuated. Similarly, a high-risk pool subsidized by others also weakens the incentive to protect one's self against becoming a high risk. Depending on the parameters, there is some combination of a safety net for people who fall through the cracks and a subsidy for low-income people at all risk levels that will maximize the proportion who choose to be insured, but what is it?

A combination of guaranteed renewability requirements and a subsidy to that coverage feature (as well as the assumed subsidy to high risks) might lead to a reasonable compromise and to a solution that would not require strict regulation of low-coverage policies since there should be lessened demand for such policies in the presence of guaranteed renewability. Some people inevitably will show up as high risks without insurance, and telling them "you should have bought guaranteed renewability coverage when you had the chance" may seem too hard-hearted. The key point, however, is that this feature can substantially protect against the fatal flaw of community rating. But what if we do not want to bet everything on subsidized coverage with guaranteed renewability?

There are two alternative strategies. One strategy penalizes people for being uninsured and high risk but tempers the penalty from what it would be under full risk rating for new applicants. Both rating-band regulation that allows some limited risk rating and high-risk pools that charge high risks more in the pool (or offer them less attractive coverage) are examples here. For reasons discussed earlier, high-risk pools are superior to insurance regulation as a way of providing coverage as a last resort. In these cases there is still value to guaranteed renewability, but because incentives are dissipated there may need to be requirements for it. Note that guaranteed renewability still has value, keeping people who do buy coverage (before they become high risks) out of the high-risk pool or the upper band.

The other strategy is to have strict community rating—high risks are entitled to the same premium level as all others—but penalize people for becoming high risk and uninsured by denying coverage, either through excluding high-risk conditions or by putting waiting periods or annual one-time sign-up periods on access to coverage. A feature in some of the reform bills is to forbid exclusions for people who previously had qualified coverage but permit them to some extent for people who chose to be uninsured for a time. Despite the apparently greater political appeal of these steps, especially the latter, they actually are inferior in concept to risk rating, since they compel people to remain uninsured, for some or all conditions, who might have been willing to pay enough to get coverage. That is, even though one might be willing to pay to sign up now as a high risk, under the annual enrollment model one must wait uninsured until the time comes. In principle there could be exceptions that would permit people to sign up earlier or sign up for coverage of all conditions by paying a penalty; then risk rating returns de facto and there is a value again to guaranteed renewability. Even in this case it may be hard for someone to pay more to avoid being anti-cream-skimmed or to have the option to take a more limited coverage plan. The situation is bound to be confusing and uncomfortable for buyers and insurers alike.

There is a system that is better than community rating and regulation prohibiting exclusions; there is a better way to achieve the same goals. Here is a way to think about what a reformed system might look like that makes some reasonable compromises but still relies on guaranteed renewability and insurer competition to drive costs and coverage. Think of the two parts of the population: those with high enough incomes that subsidies beyond a minimal level are both unneeded and unjust, versus those with lower incomes who need help to obtain insurance at any risk level.

The higher-income part of the population should be incentivized (through a mandate or penalty) to get catastrophic insurance with guaranteed renewability. Coverage can be sought from any source (employment-based group, exchange, individual market) the consumer finds attractive. All policies regardless of source would be guaranteed renewable at class average premiums for the individual insured. Policy specifications should be clarified and made transparent, and unreasonable pre-existing-condition provisions—the kind no one would buy if they were careful—should be excluded. Exchanges might be made available as an option. Beyond these minimal steps, the market could be left free to function for the bulk of the population.

For those for whom low income or large family size prompts a social desire for more generous subsidies, those subsidies should be offered in the form of vouchers, with qualified coverage specified as parsimoniously as possible (and also taking the form of catastrophic coverage, but the out-of-pocket maximum described as catastrophic linked to income). The same modest rules about guaranteed renewability and policy transparency would also apply.

For the small fraction of people who somehow do not have guaranteed renewability protection and who are above-average risk, the value of the credit would be augmented somewhat but the generosity of the policy would be limited; the person who falls into this situation would pay more and get less than if they had bought and retained guaranteed renewable coverage. Insurers could charge full risk-based premiums to this population but the credit would be risk-adjusted to some extent to cushion the impact on the portion of the premium the consumer would have to pay.

If political pressure and/or administrative convenience dictated some limits on risk rating of premiums, those limits would be modest in amount and would apply to coverage for which only a small fraction of the population—those who are high risks and without health insurance—would be eligible. Similar modest limits would be placed on any efforts to constrain exclusion provisions that consumers found attractive as a way to hold down premiums and deal with adverse selection.

Conclusion

I have not considered all possible improvements in the individual market here. The amount of even reasonably definitive information on the comparative performance of these devices is currently quite low, and so there is little benefit from going into great detail about what it is we do not know.

In my judgment, the policy that follows from this frank admission of imperfect information is one that might be sensible in any case: the optimal government intervention is one that provides appropriate subsidies to those who need them, a basic but initially quite limited regulatory framework, the possibility for a large number of different qualified sources of insurance—for-profit and nonprofit, public and private—and then permits consumers to make their own choices in a neutral way. If higher-income people who remain uninsured are thought to be a policy problem (rather than as evidence that not all rich people are smart), a penalty or mandate might be considered. Should additional subsidies and regulations be required, they can more easily be added when needed than withdrawn if not needed.

For good reasons, reform of the individual health insurance market is on the front burner in today's policy kitchen. But the recipe for reform in currently proposed legislation is far from ideal and stands a good chance of making things worse rather than better. It would run a real risk of increasing the number of uninsured (given subsidies offered), stifling innovation in health insurance at a time when it is most needed, and creating dysfunctional incentives for both consumers and insurance companies. Reform which uses rather than abuses market forces would be preferable. Competitive markets do have their strongest rationale in settings in which the amount of knowledge a planner has or could have is incomplete, and the individual health insurance market is a prime candidate for such a setting. There are some serious trade-offs between different policy features, but the model of open, neutral competitive markets seems best suited to having those trade-offs made as well as they can be in the world in which we now live.

References

America's Health Insurance Plans. *A Comprehensive Survey of Premiums, Availability and Benefits, 2006–2007.* AHIP. December 2007.

Austin, D. Andrew, and Thomas L. Hungerford. "The Market Structure of the Health Insurance Industry." Congressional Research Service report for Congress, October 15, 2009.

Baker, Charlie. "Small Group Reform in Massachusetts." *Let's Talk Healthcare.* Blog. May 18, 2009. http://www.letstalkhealthcare.org/uncategoized/small-group-reform-in-massachusetts (accessed November 12, 2009).

Beeuwkes Buntin, Melinda, M. Susan Marquis, and Jill M. Yegian. "The Role of the Individual Health Insurance Market: Prospects for Change." *Health Affairs* 23, no. 6 (2004): 79–90.

Bluhm, William. "Duration-based Policy Reserves." *Transactions of the Society of Actuaries* 19, no. 3 (2006): 11–32.

———. *Individual Health Insurance.* Winstead, CT: ACTEX Publishing, 2007.

Bundorf, M. Kate, Bradley J. Herring, and Mark V. Pauly. "Health Risk, Income, and Employment-Based Health Insurance." *Forum for Health Economics and Policy,* forthcoming.

Chollet, D. S., and A. M. Kirk. *Understanding Individual*

Health Insurance Markets: Standards, Practices, and Products in Ten States. Washington, D.C.: Alpha Center, 1998.

Cochrane, John. "Time-Consistent Health Insurance." *Journal of Political Economy* 103, no. 3 (1995): 445–73.

Commonwealth Fund. "2007 Biennial Survey of Health Insurance." 2009. http://www.commonwealthfund.org/Content/Grants/2006/Dec/The-Commonwealth-Fund-2007-Biennial-Health-Insurance-Survey.aspx (accessed October 29, 2009).

Frakt, Austin B., Steven Pizer, and Marian Vrobel. "High Risk Pools for Uninsurable Individuals: Recent Growth, Future Prospects." *Health Care Financing Review* 26.2 (2004): 73–85.

Herring, Bradley J., and Mark V. Pauly. "Risk Pooling and Regulation: Policy and Reality in Today's Individual Health Insurance Market." *Health Affairs* 26.3 (2007): 770–79.

Holtz-Eakin, Douglas. *Washington Week in Review.* October 29, 2007.

Kingsdale, Jon, and John M. Bertko. "Health Insurance Exchanges: A Typology and Guide to Key Design Issues." *Health Industry Forum.* July 20, 2009.

Kunreuther, Howard C., Mark V. Pauly, and Stacey McMorrow. *Anomalies in Insurance Markets.* Cambridge University Press, forthcoming.

Marquis, M. Susan, et al. "Consumer Decision Making in the Individual Health Insurance Market." *Health Affairs* 25.3 (2006): w226–w234. http://content.healthaffairs.org/cgi/reprint/25/3/w226 (accessed August 28, 2009).

National Association of Health Underwriters. "Cost and Availability of Insurance for People with Chronic Health Conditions." Press release, March 12, 2002.

Newhouse, Joseph P., and the Insurance Experiment Study

Group. *Free for All? Lessons from the Rand Health Insurance Experiment.* Cambridge, MA: Harvard University Press, 1993.

Patel, Vip, and Mark V. Pauly. "Guaranteed Renewability and the Problem of Risk Variation in Individual Health Insurance Markets." *Health Affairs* 21.4 (2002): w280–w289. http://content.healthaffairs.org/cgi/reprint/hlthaff.w2.280v1 (accessed October 29, 2009).

Pauly, Mark V. "The Economics of Moral Hazard." *American Economic Review* 58 (1968): 531–537.

———. "The Welfare Economics of Community Rating." *Journal of Risk and Insurance* (1970): 310–21.

———. *Health Benefits at Work.* Ann Arbor: University of Michigan Press, 1997.

———. "Risks and Benefits in Health Care." *Health Affairs* 26.3 (2007): 653–62.

———. "Adverse Selection and Moral Hazard: Implications for Health Insurance Markets." *Incentives and Choice in Health and Health Care.* Eds. Frank A. Sloan and Hirschel Kasper. Cambridge, MA: MIT Press, 2008. 103–129.

Pauly, Mark V., and Bradley J. Herring. *Pooling Health Insurance Risk.* Washington, DC: AEI Press, 1999.

———. "Incentive-compatible Guaranteed Renewable Health Insurance Premiums." *Journal of Health Economics* 25.3 (2006): 395–417.

Pauly, Mark V., Bradley J. Herring, and David K. Song. "Information Technology and Consumer Search for Health Insurance." *The International Journal of the Economics of Business* 13.1 (2006): 45–63.

Pauly, Mark V., et al. "Competitive Behavior in the HMO Marketplace." *Health Affairs* 21.1 (2002): 194–202.

Pauly, Mark V., Howard Kunreuther, and Richard Hirth. "Guaranteed Renewability in Insurance." *Journal of Risk and Uncertainty* 10.2 (1995): 143–56.

Pauly, Mark V., and Robert Lieberthal. "How Risky Is Individual Health Insurance?" *Health Affairs* 27.3 (2008): w242–w249. http://content.healthaffairs.org/cgi/reprint/27/3/w242 (accessed August 28, 2009).

Pauly, Mark V., Allison Percy, and Bradley J. Herring. "Individual versus Job-Based Health Insurance: Weighing the Pros and Cons." *Health Affairs* 18.6 (1999): 28–44.

Pollitz, Karen, and Richard Sorian. "How Accessible Is Individual Health Insurance for Consumers in Less Than Perfect Health?" Kaiser Family Foundation, 2001.

Sheiner, Louise. *Health Care Costs, Wages, and Aging.* Federal Reserve Board of Governors, Finance and Economics Discussion Series, no. 1999–19. Washington, DC: FRB, 1999.

Sood, Neeraj, et al. "Health Insurance: Should California Regulate Health Insurance Premiums?" Rand Corporation, 2004.

Sunstein, Cass R., and Richard H. Thaler. *Nudge: Improving Decisions about Health, Wealth, and Happiness.* New York: Penguin Books, 2008.

Swartz, K., and D. W. Garnick. "Lessons from New Jersey." *Journal of Health Politics, Policy, and Law* 25.1 (February 2000): 45–70.

Turnbull, Nancy. Comment on "What's the Role of a Health Exchange?" in *Let's Talk Healthcare.* Blog by Charlie Baker. July 9, 2009. http://www.letstalkhealthcare.org/ma-health-reform/whats-the-role-of-a-health-exchange/ (accessed November 12, 2009).

Yegian, Jill M., et al. "The Nonpoor Uninsured in California, 1998." *Health Affairs* 19.4 (2000): 171–77.

About the Author

MARK V. PAULY holds the position of Bendheim Professor in the Department of Health Care Systems at the
Wharton School of the University of Pennsylvania. He
received a PhD in economics from the University of Vir-
ginia. He is a professor of health-care systems, insurance
and risk management, and business and public policy at
the Wharton School and professor of economics in the
School of Arts and Sciences at the University of Pennsylvania. Professor Pauly is a former commissioner on the
Physician Payment Review Commission and an active
member of the Institute of Medicine. One of the nation's
leading health economists, Pauly has made significant
contributions to the fields of medical economics and
health insurance. His classic study on the economics of
moral hazard was the first to point out how health insurance coverage may affect patients' use of medical services. Subsequent work, both theoretical and empirical,
has explored the effect of conventional insurance coverage on preventive care, on outpatient care, and on pre-
scription drug use in managed care. He is currently
studying the effect of poor health on worker productiv-

ity. In addition, he has explored the influences that de-termine whether insurance coverage is available and, through several cost-effectiveness studies, the influence of medical care and health practices on health outcomes and cost. His work in health policy deals with the ap-propriate design for Medicare in a budget-constrained environment and the ways to reduce the number of un-insured through tax credits for public and private insur-ance. Pauly is coeditor in chief of the *International Journal of Health Care, Finance, and Economics* and associate editor of the *Journal of Risk and Uncertainty.* He has served on the Institute of Medicine panels on improving the financing of vaccines and on public ac-countability for health insurers under Medicare. He is an appointed member of the U.S. Department of Health and Human Services National Advisory Committee to the Agency for Healthcare Research and Quality.

WORKING GROUP ON
HEALTH CARE POLICY

HOOVER
INSTITUTION
STANFORD
UNIVERSITY

The WORKING GROUP ON HEALTH CARE POLICY will aim to devise public policies that enable more Americans to get better value for their health care dollar and foster appropriate innovation that extends and improves life. Key principles that guide policy formation include the central role of individual choice and competitive markets in financing and delivering health services, individual responsibility for health behaviors and decisions, and appropriate guidelines for government intervention in health care markets.

The core membership of this working group includes Scott W. Atlas, John F. Cogan, R. Glenn Hubbard, Daniel P. Kessler, Mark V. Pauly, and Charles E. Phelps.

Index